COPYRIGHT PAGE

ISBN 13: 9781731562272

© 2018 Shawn Beaton All Rights Reserved

Scripture taken from the New King James Version®. Copyright © 1982 by Thomas Nelson. Used by permission. All rights reserved.

THE HOLY BIBLE, NEW INTERNATIONAL VERSION®, NIV® Copyright © 1973, 1978, 1984, 2011 by Biblica, Inc.® Used by permission. All rights reserved worldwide.

Cover Images from www.shutterstock.com

By Melinda Nagy

Royalty-free stock photo ID: 1231649860
cheering crowd watching fireworks - new year concept

By Head_Snake

Royalty-free stock photo ID: 1226836903
Hypomelanistic Burmese python

TABLE OF CONTENTS

Introduction 4

Ancient History Relating to the Python Spirit 7

Python the Slave Master 9

A Study of the Python Spirit and Philippi in the Book of Acts 14

Python's Manipulation of Stock Markets and the News Cycles 28

Python's Use of Hate, Fear and Intoxicants to Create Mob Violence 38

The Python Spirit and its Religion of Rebellion. 46

The Python Spirit's Role in Mental Illness, Sicknesses, Drug Addiction, Prisons and Medicine 57

Python's Use of False Prophecy and Witchcraft Today 69

How to Defeat Python 88

Donald Trump the Destroyer 102

Introduction

During the writing of this book God showed me an encouraging sign that it was no mistake I was writing this book and that the Church of Jesus Christ was getting victory over the python spirit. In the state of Florida, a man captured a record setting 17+ foot python!ⁱ This took place on November 5, 2018. The reason why I believe this is a sign to the Church of Jesus Christ is the name of the man who captured this python. His name is Kyle Penniston. The meaning of the name Kyle is "church" in the Gaelic language. In addition, this man made a statement which I believe is prophetic. He said, "So this snake just showed me you really can do anything."ⁱⁱ The reason why I believe this is prophetic is because it sounds very similar to what Paul the Apostle wrote to the church of Philippi, *"I can do all things through Christ who strengthens me"*, (Philippians 4:13 NKJV). Philippi was the city where Paul met the spirit of python inside a slave girl (Acts 16:16) and he undoubtedly wrote the above verse to encourage this city church. Paul's encounter with the python spirit was not easy as it harassed him, and ultimately had him tortured and imprisoned. Like the python in the natural the python spirit is very strong and will try very hard to squeeze the life and hope out of any person. It is only through the strength Jesus Christ supplies that we can overpower the python spirit. This man Kyle Penniston apparently came close to being overpowered by the python but managed to euthanize it. This python thought it would kill this man, but the python was the one that ended up dying. Likewise, the python spirit believes it will kill many of you reading this book, but you will bring about its death through the strength of Jesus Christ!

Within this book you will discover the true nature of the python spirit. This spirit leads a religion of rebellion and convinces people they are free when they are in reality slaves. It is for this reason I confront the issue of rebellion within and without the Church. This spirit is very rebellious, and the reason for why it is so strong. The python spirit will not be defeated through binding alone, but also through repenting of the sin of rebellion. There is also a chapter at the end of this book that unveils how this spirit is influencing President Trump. In addition, I provide clear insight into why the world is so crazy right now and President Trump's role in reforming it or possibly bringing destruction to parts of it!

I conclude this introduction by saying that Jesus Christ is calling each one of us into a life of radical obedience. It is only through this kind of obedience that the python spirit can be completely destroyed. Do not worry for Jesus Christ will supply us with the strength we need to obey Him. It is my hope that you experience the strength of Jesus Christ surging through you as you read this book and that you find freedom from any prison the python spirit may have thrown you into.

LET THE WEAK SAY,

'I AM STRONG.'

JOEL 3:10b NKJV

Ancient History Relating to the Python Spirit

I do not want to go into great detail about the origins of the python spirit because it is rooted in mythology. But there is some basic knowledge about this spirit and how it operates through the tales surrounding it. In ancient Greece there was a location called the oracle of Delphi. At this place was a temple dedicated to the god Apollo where it was believed that the priestesses of Apollo would fall into a trance and prophesy while they were under the influence of gases coming from a fissure in the surface of the earth. A legend provides the reason for these gases coming from the fissure to be caused by the rotting corpse of a large serpent or dragon. The legend tells us that a large serpent or dragon dwelt in the center of the earth but was killed by the god Apollo in revenge for it harassing a relative of his. When Apollo killed this python, its rotting corpse is supposed to have created the fumes coming from the crack in the earth. It would appear that the god Apollo and the python spirit are almost married to one another. The fumes of the python are reputed to have given these priestesses of Apollo their divinatory powers, but the god Apollo was also known as a god of prophecy himself. It is likely that the worship of Apollo replaced the worship of the python, but in reality, they are one and the same. It is for this reason diviners in ancient Greece were known to have a spirit of python.

I believe this brief overview of the myth behind the origins of the python spirit are sufficient as I do not want to glorify Greek mythology in anyway but steer you the reader towards the Bible!

And it came to pass as we were going to prayer that a certain female slave, having a spirit of Python, met us, who brought much profit to her masters by prophesying.   **Acts 16:16**

Python the Slave Master

When people think of the python spirit, they generally regard this spirit as a spirit of divination. This is true for most translations translate python to "divination". But I believe the true nature of this spirit is missed. It is my conviction that the spirit of python is primarily a spirit of enslavement. Divination or witchcraft is one of many ways this spirit enslaves mankind.

Now it happened, as we went to prayer, that a certain slave girl possessed with a spirit of divination met us, who brought her masters much profit by fortune-telling. This girl followed Paul and us, and cried out, saying, "These men are the servants of the Most High God, who proclaim to us the way of salvation." And this she did for many days.

Acts 16:16-18a NKJV

These verses give us a lot of clues as to why the python spirit is an enslaving spirit and not merely a spirit of divination. First of all, we can see that the victim of this spirit of divination/python is a slave. The victim is not only a slave, but a girl. This reminds me of the modern-day sex slave industry. Many young girls and women are prisoners of this spirit and reside in prisons of lust. These girls/women are given drugs to further enslave them and keep them dependent on their slave master. Slavery and drugs are very much connected. In a later chapter we will examine how the python spirit uses narcotics to enslave millions.

This girl is described as being "possessed". Possession implies ownership and we see that the girl's true master was the python spirit and not her human masters. Possession is the ultimate goal of this spirit. This spirit loves to mimic the Holy Spirit and possess unbelievers and believers alike, however, this spirit cannot possess a believer because they have been purchased by the shed blood of Jesus Christ and are sealed by the Holy Spirit!

And you also were included in Christ when you heard the message of truth, the gospel of salvation. When you believed, you were marked in him with a seal, the promised Holy Spirit, who is a deposit guaranteeing our inheritance until the remembrance of those who are God's possession—to the praise of his glory.

Ephesians 1:13-14 NIV

Fortunately, the python spirit cannot possess believers in Jesus Christ, but they can be enslaved by it through witchcraft, drugs, depression and many other avenues. Any new believer may struggle in some of these areas that enslaved them in their prior life and battle with doubts concerning their salvation. This enslavement is used by the python spirit to discourage the believer in Jesus Christ in an attempt to make them doubt they belong to Jesus Christ. The believer in Jesus

Christ is a child of God, but they will need deliverance from demons. When the python spirit and other demons are cast out the believer they will experience greater freedom and confidence of their salvation. In the meantime, the believer in Jesus Christ must remember when they first heard and believed the gospel of Jesus Christ. This moment is precious and marks the time we were sealed with the Holy Spirit. When we were sealed by the Holy Spirit we became the possession of God and our salvation is secure! Reread the two verses I posted above from Ephesians if you need encouragement.

Going back to the verses of Acts 16:16-18 we can see this girl followed Paul and his companions for many days and cried out they were servants of God. We can also see the enslaving nature of this spirit as it continually compelled this girl to follow them and repeatedly proclaim the same thing about Paul and his friends. When the python spirit is at work in a person they will find themselves bound by addictions or a ritualistic behavior which takes on a religious fervor of sorts. There are many who struggle with obsessions and compulsions of various kinds. Like this girl some are bound with an obsession for certain persons and stalk them. The goal of this stalking behavior is control of the victim being stalked. This spirit will try to enslave others through its host and manipulate their target with fear, mind games and sexually aggressive behavior aided by spirits of lust.

She followed Paul and the rest of us, shouting, "These men are servants of the Most High God, who are telling you the way to be saved."

Acts 16:17 NIV

Another important feature of this passage in the book of Acts is the matter of this girl with the spirit of python recognizing that Paul and his companions are servants of God. Paul and his companions were heading to a place of prayer. This is one of the ways Paul and his companions served God. The title of servant basically means slave. God calls us to serve Him or become His bond servants. The spirit of python did not want Paul and his friends to serve God but become enslaved to the harassment of it. Harassment can distract us and make us unable focus on our service to God. This spirit did not want them to be focused on prayer but caught up in the celebrity they were receiving through the promotional activity of this spirit. This spirit does the same today keeping people busy with social media and speaking engagements. At first popularity seems appealing, but it eventually becomes an all-consuming preoccupation. Some neglect a personal relationship with Jesus Christ through prayer and choose to focus on the celebrity of being a megachurch pastor. If one is not careful they can begin to serve the spirit of python and not God. Whatever we serve becomes our master.

It is believed that the city of Philippi where this slave girl and Paul encountered each other was composed primarily of slaves.[iii] Wherever this spirit is operating there will be some kind of slavery at work. When literal slavery is not taking place, it will generally be creating mental slaves. In many organizations today, individual opinion is not encouraged, however, conformity is applauded. This has taken place in the workplace, culture and government through political correctness. Nothing unique comes out of these places anymore because everyone is a clone repeating the same message of the CEO or leader. Some may desire to express their opinion or break out of this uniformity, but they are kept in line through fear. Political correctness has silenced many through fear of punishment and created a society of slaves.

A Study of the Python Spirit and Philippi in the Book of Acts

Therefore, sailing from Troas, we ran a straight course to Samothrace, and the next day came to Neapolis, and from there to Philippi, which is the foremost city of that part of Macedonia, a colony. And on the Sabbath day we went out of the city to the riverside, where prayer was customarily made; and we sat down and spoke to the women who met there.

Acts 16:11-13 NKJV

Here we are introduced to the city of Philippi. When people generally look at the spirit of python they begin with its introduction at verse 16. But the verses preceding verse 16 give us clues about the culture of the city of Philippi this spirit ruled over.

Looking at the verses above I believe we are seeing some form of segregation at work. These women were praying outside the city and no men seem to be present besides Paul and his companions who are visiting the city. When slavery is present there is generally some form of segregation at work also. We have already seen the girl slave with the spirit of python in verse 16. It is my belief that women had few to no rights in the city of Philippi. Throughout the Roman world women generally had few rights and were often treated no better than slaves.[iv]

In the New Age movement many of its members are women. Women are led to believe that witchcraft is their key to becoming equal or throwing off the oppression of male misogyny. But the spirit of python that controls witchcraft has no interest in the freedom of women and is working towards their enslavement. Unfortunately, many women are led to believe there is no role for women in the Church because the Church throughout history has often discouraged women from participating in the Church or even working a job. Women were often reduced to a servile role and one who gave birth to children and reared them. There is nothing evil about serving and being a traditional stay at home mom, but Jesus Christ calls some women to run their own businesses and to participate in church ministry. I am not interested in debating what roles women are to play in the Church or society, but I do know that it is more than what they had throughout history.

Jesus Christ wants to speak through women as much as men. There is no preferred gender when it comes to prophesying. The spirit of python is a spirit of divination or false prophecy. It wants women to believe they have no voice in the Church, but this is a lie. In fact, women were often seen playing a prophetic role in the Church and the Old Testament.

On the next day we who were Paul's companions departed and came to Caesarea, and entered the

house of Philipp the evangelist, who was one of the seven, and stayed with him. Now this man had four virgin daughters who prophesied. And as we stayed many days, a certain prophet named Agabus came down from Judea.

Acts 21:8-10 NKJV

Later in the book of Acts we see the companions of Paul visiting Philipp the Evangelist. Coincidentally, Philipp's name is similar to Philippi. Philipp has four daughters who prophesied and there is mention of a prophet named Agabus. In the Old Testament there were women prophets such as Miriam and Deborah. Therefore, a woman need not become a witch to have a voice on spiritual matters but can prophesy in the Church and possibly become a prophet. At the same time I want to remind any reader the Church is not a place for those seeking notoriety and authority, but for those who seek to bring glory to Jesus Christ!

The spirit of python wants to enslave people if he can, but the Holy Spirit wants to bring us freedom. I find it interesting these women and Paul's group are meeting outside the city by the riverside. This reminds me of the need for some who have the need to leave the traditional Church to find freedom. I'm not talking about apostasy here, but many churches are so steeped in traditions that they do not permit women or others to have a voice in the Church of Jesus Christ. Some will need to find a church where they can serve and have a voice. The Holy Spirit is often represented as a river or rivers. A river must flow freely and not be dammed up.

Now the Lord is the Spirit; and where the Spirit of the Lord is, there is liberty.

2 Corinthians 3:17 NKJV

When the Church thinks of groups they need to evangelize they often think in terms of racial or language groups. But the need to evangelize women or men with the gospel of Jesus Christ is just as important! In some regions of the earth a particular gender may be under the domination of Satan. In the city of Philippi, it appears that the women in particular were under the domination of the python spirit. Fortunately, Paul and his friends were able to evangelize a woman who had her own business. Unlike the slave girl this woman was not someone else's property but owned her own business. I believe this believer is a model for some woman to aspire to.

Now a certain woman named Lydia heard us. She was a seller of purple from the city of Thyatira, who worshiped God. The Lord opened her heart to heed the things spoken by Paul. And when she and her household were baptized, she begged us, saying, "If you have judged me to be faithful to the Lord, come to my house and stay." So she persuaded us.

Acts 16:14-15 NKJV

Ironically society has changed a great deal today and many would feel that men as a gender are under attack. While men are respected better within the Church they are generally hated in society in throughout the culture of the Western world. It has become such an epidemic that movie sequels or new movies are created with an all female cast or few men in it. The purpose is to replace men and redefine who is in control of society. It is for this reason that any church doing spiritual warfare must see which groups whether they be a gender, or a race are under attack the most. Spiritual warfare can be more precise with this knowledge.

In a later chapter we will look at false prophets, but we must touch on it here. One of the methods by which the spirit of python works is to speak through a false prophet and promote a race, gender or group above all others while demonizing others. This creates an atmosphere of division and segregation. I am not against a majority rule and I would endorse it in most cases, but when the majority or a favored group begin to hate, persecute and kill another it is demonic.

Now it happened, as we went to prayer, that a certain slave girl possessed with a spirit of divination met us, who brought her masters much profit by fortune-telling. This girl followed Paul and us, and cried out, saying, "These men are servants of the Most High God, who proclaim to us the way of salvation." And

this she did for many days. But Paul, greatly annoyed, turned and said to the spirit, "I command you in the name of Jesus Christ to come out of her." And he came out that very hour.

Acts 16:16-18 NKJV

When Paul and his companions began to pray in the region of Philippi it started to change the atmosphere. This is good, but it also exposed the ruling power of the city. In this case it was the spirit of divination or python. Divination is the same as witchcraft and it represents false spiritual authority for it opposes the authority of God's kingdom. When I was doing research on the python spirit and the city of Philippi I discovered that the city had no synagogue. I find this surprising considering Philippi was one of the foremost cities in Macedonia according to Acts 16:12. In Acts 16:16-18 we see that Paul and his companions were continually harassed by the slave girl with the spirit of divination or python. Considering the fact that there was no synagogue in Philippi, that prayer was made outside the city and the continual harassment of this python spirit we can conclude that this spirit had a firm control over spiritual matters in the city. The spirit of python or divination is not like any other spirit ruling a city. The python spirit is very controlling and resistant to change for its power is rooted in rebellion!

For rebellion is like the sin of divination, and arrogance like the evil of idolatry. Because you have

rejected the word of the Lord, he has rejected you as king."

1 Samuel 15:23 NIV

Have you ever noticed how hard it is to change someone's opinion or culture? The reason why it is so hard to share Jesus Christ with people or change the culture of an area is rebellion. The root of most sin is rebellion and most people won't repent of sin until the root sin of rebellion is dealt with. We can see how resistant this python spirit was for it followed and harassed Paul and his friends many days. I imagine Paul and his friends must have prayed for this girl many times if she was harassing them several days. Nothing seemed to change until Paul cast the spirit out of the girl when he had enough of being annoyed by this spirit. But this did not end the persecution for Paul and his companions would suffer much more.

When her owners realized that their hope of making money was gone, they seized Paul and Silas and dragged them into the marketplace to face the authorities. They brought them before the magistrates and said, "These men are Jews, and are throwing our city into an uproar by advocating customs unlawful for us Romans to accept or practice."

Acts 16:19-21 NIV

Just as the python spirit attempted to manipulate Paul and his companions through harassment it was now trying to manipulate the magistrates against them. The owners/masters representing the python spirit dragged Paul and his friends before these magistrates. They are angry with their teaching and the loss of their profits. The python spirit hates the freedom of speech and wants to suffocate the voices of truth and freedom. These masters mention the ethnicity of Paul and his friends which was totally unnecessary and make a judgement on the religious customs they followed which was ridiculous considering these people followed many different gods. Like our modern-day system of political correctness, we see there was tolerance for everything but Christianity.

The crowd joined in the attack against Paul and Silas, and the magistrates ordered them to be stripped and beaten with rods. After they had been severely flogged, they were thrown into prison, and the jailer was commanded to guard them carefully. When he received these orders, he put them in the inner cell and fastened their feet in the stocks.

Acts 16:22-24 NIV

Like the fake news of today the python spirit controlled public opinion and turned the people against Paul and his companions and their Christian message. Fortunately, public opinion is turning against the fake news of our day, but it didn't happen overnight. But nations like the United States are still very divided between those who believe the fake news/political correctness and those who do not. Slowly the fear of punishment used by political correctness to silence and cower Christians is being broken. Paul and Silas were beaten and flogged as a lesson not to propagate the Christian message anymore and to discourage anyone else considering the Christian faith as a lifestyle. We can see the spirit of divination/python is primarily concerned with controlling and enslaving a people. It will use harassment, witchcraft, violent persecution and mental illness in an effort to break the Christian.

I wonder if Paul and his companions were prayer walking throughout the city. Some teachers have suggested that prayer walking is a powerful form of spiritual warfare and a way to take the Church into the community. We know Paul and his companions were going to prayer at the time of the confrontation between Paul and the python spirit. Therefore, it is not surprising that the feet of Paul and Silas were fastened in stocks. Remember the slave girl with the python spirit followed Paul and his companions for several days. Paul's group must've been preaching and praying throughout the city of Philippi. Observe how Paul and Silas become very much like the slave girl and are locked up in an inner cell. This python spirit wanted to control them and prevent their ministry throughout the city. The issue of control is always present when this spirit is in operation. Fortunately, Paul and Silas refused to be controlled and continued in their prayers to God.

About midnight Paul and Silas were praying and singing hymns to God, and the other prisoners were listening to them. Suddenly there was such a violent earthquake that the foundations of the prison were shaken. At once all the prison doors flew open, and everyone's chains came loose. The jailer woke up, and when he saw the prison doors open, he drew his sword and was about to kill himself because he thought the prisoners had escaped. But Paul shouted, "Don't harm yourself! We are all here!"

Acts 16:25-28 NIV

In the above verses we see Paul and Silas overcome the depression and hopelessness the python spirit was trying to bring upon them by continuing to do what got them in trouble in the first place! Paul and Silas refused to despair and continued their ministry of prayer in the prison. This is a good lesson for every Christian. The enemy cannot control our attitude or perspective of our situation. Our environment does not determine whether we are victorious or not, but our faith in Jesus Christ does! Paul and Silas are praying to Jesus Christ and worshipping Him at midnight when night is darkest. Midnight can represent the last days. In a later chapter we will look at how this spirit will fight the

Church in the last days before the return of Jesus Christ. The overcoming faith of Paul and Silas defies their dark prison and results in liberation through Jesus Christ in the form of a violent earthquake. This must've been a joyous moment for Paul and his fellow prisoners, but not for the jailer who has awoke. He likely feared death or torture for his failure to keep the prisoners imprisoned and decides to commit suicide. In the following verses we will see that this jailer had a serious issue with depression and his decision to commit suicide was strongly influenced by this. The python spirit is strongly involved in mental health issues and will try to make things appear hopeless as its squeezes the hope and life out of a person. Many have committed suicide because of the python spirit.

The jailer called for lights, rushed in and fell trembling before Paul and Silas. He then brought them out and asked, "Sirs, what must I do to be saved?" They replied, "Believe in the Lord Jesus, and you will be saved—you and your household." Then they spoke the word of the Lord to him and to all the others in his house. At that hour of the night the jailer took them and washed their wounds; then immediately he and all his household were baptized. The jailer brought them into his house and set a meal before them; he was filled with joy because he had come to believe in God—he and his whole household.

Acts 16:29-34 NIV

I find it interesting that the jailer runs in with lights to investigate what has become of the jail and the prisoners after the quake. I believe it symbolizes a revelation of Jesus Christ and hope. Before Jesus Christ enters our lives, we will live in spiritual darkness and a state of hopelessness. Like the jail Paul and Silas were in there is a prison of a depressed and hopeless mind. This jailer was bound by the python spirit, but the earthquake that God sent not only freed the prisoners, but the jailer and his household. They were able to receive Jesus Christ as their savior. Like the prison holding Paul and Silas it takes tremendous power to defeat the python spirit in an individual's life or region. Hopelessness and depression can be stubborn companions when the python spirit is around, but Jesus Christ can save us from the python spirit or any other demon of hell! When the jailer receives Jesus Christ along with his family he begins to experience joy. Like the feet of Paul and Silas being physically bound some are spiritually bound in their feet by the python spirit. There is no spring in the steps of these victims or any kind of joy. They go throughout life drudging along, but when they are freed from the python spirit, they feel alive! In a later chapter we will look at how the python spirit is involved in depression.

And when it was day, the magistrates sent the officers, saying, "Let those men go." So the keeper of the prison reported these words to Paul, saying, "The magistrates have sent to let you go. Now therefore

depart, and go in peace." But Paul said to them, "They have beaten us openly, uncondemned Romans, and have thrown us into prisons. And now do they put us out secretly? No indeed! Let them come themselves and get us out." And the officers told these words to the magistrates, and they were afraid when they heard that they were Romans. Then they came and pleaded with them and brought them out, and asked them to depart from the city. So they went out of the prison and entered the house of Lydia; and when they had seen the brethren, they encouraged them and departed.

Acts 16:35-40 NKJV

The python spirit has just been humbled in the city of Philippi and those he rules through. But like the fake news of today they did not want the public to know they had been humbled. Even after defeat the python spirit wanted to control how things appeared and to project the idea he was still in control through these magistrates. But Paul nor Jesus Christ was going to allow such a deception. The magistrates had to come to Paul and Silas and apologize for beating them as they were Roman citizens. Roman citizens had certain rights throughout the empire and could not be tortured. The python spirit likes to silence and isolate Christians in prisons both literal and social. It wants Christians and others to believe they have no rights and to ignore Christian persecution in our nation or the world. It desires to ostracize the believer, but we must not allow this to happen. An injustice was done to Paul and Silas and they demanded an apology. Likewise, Christians cannot be afraid to fight for their rights or to get justice. We cannot allow the python spirit to control the news cycle or the dialogue circulating in the community. It wants to choke out our voice, but we must resist and be loud! We should listen to organizations like the Voice of the Martyrs[v] who keep us informed about Christian persecution. It seems like many in the government, media and the NGO community are rarely concerned with the persecution of Christians or Jews for that matter. I believe it is important to support Christian organizations who are advocating for the freedom of persecuted Christians or that are lobbying our governments for Christian rights and freedoms.

Python's Manipulation of Stock Markets and the News Cycles

It is obvious that the python spirit is involved in divination, but it is also involved in the financial world. Since the python spirit is primarily concerned with the enslavement of mankind its needs to be involved in the one of the greatest tools of slavery which is money. When we think of spirits connected with money we generally think of Mammon. But money or Mammon is subordinate to the python spirit and it manipulates this whole system. In the final world empire, we see how the python spirit will use money to enslave all of mankind!

Then I saw another beast coming up out of the earth, and he had two horns like a lamb and spoke like a dragon. And he exercises all the authority of the first beast in his presence, and causes the earth and those who dwell in it to worship the first beast, whose deadly wound was healed. He performs great signs, so that he even makes fire come down from heaven on the earth in the sight of men. And he deceives those who dwell on the earth by those signs which he was granted to do in the sight of the beast, telling those who dwell on the earth to make an image to the beast who was wounded by the sword and lived. He was granted power to give breath to the image of the beast, that the image of the beast should speak and

cause as many as would not worship the image of the beast to be killed. He causes all, both small and great, rich and poor, free and slave, to receive a mark on their right hand or on their foreheads, and that no one may buy or sell except one who has the mark or the name of the beast, or the number of his name. Here is wisdom. Let him who has understanding calculate the number of the beast, for it is the number of a man: His number is 666.

Revelation 13:11- 18 NKJV

This second beast in the book of Revelation is often referred to as the false prophet. The spirit of divination or python oversees most false prophecy and false prophets. In this passage of Scripture, we can see that this false prophet will beguile most people with lying wonders so that they will take a mark showing their allegiance to the antichrist. By doing so all who take the mark are declaring they are the property of the antichrist. As an added incentive nobody will be able to buy or sell unless they have this mark. This essentially removes their freedom and makes them slaves.

The history of the city of Philippi shows us another reason why this spirit was attracted to this city. The city of Philippi before the time of the Roman empire was known to have gold mines nearby and the city had a mint as a result.[vi] It is my personal belief that the python spirit likes to control currency and riches as a tool to manipulate the masses.

It is my belief that Wall Street and other stock exchanges are manipulated a great deal by the python spirit. This spirit is behind the dramatic highs and lows of the stock market. These highs and lows are more about investor confidence or anxiety than actual economics. This was most evident in the roaring 20's and the Great Depression of the 30's which ultimately led to World War 2. That's how python works on a person and society. At first there is euphoria or overconfidence followed by horrible depression. Many are destroyed when the depression comes and never recover. People are literally enslaved by worry and constantly watch their stocks. Even value investing has a predictive nature to it. Is it natural talent or spirits like the python who decide winners and losers? I'm sure that many who are rich are receiving their predictive abilities from the python spirit. Predictive ability either comes from the Holy Spirit or the python spirit. Many executives and those who trade on the stock market consult psychics these days.[vii] The stock markets often see bubbles and then burst. There is always a correction because pride or euphoria goes before a fall (Proverbs 16:18).

When Donald Trump was elected president the stock market began to surge and has until now, but signs of a crash or big correction are evident in the fall of 2018. I personally would advise against investing in the stock market at this time as the Dow Jones is showing signs of great instability and big losses are coming. The reason for this is Donald Trump's decision to endorse a two-state solution on Israel on September 26, 2018.[viii] Since his endorsement of the two-state solution two dramatic warnings came to America and President Trump. On October 10, 2018 the stock market fell over 800 points[ix] and Hurricane Michael devastated the U.S. Airforce by severely damaging the Tyndall Airforce Base in Florida.[x] This reminds me of 9/11 when both the World Trade Center and Pentagon were attacked by terrorists. It is as if God is saying, "I will strike your military and economy America if you continue down this path of trying to divide Israel." On October 28, 2018 a man entered a synagogue in Pittsburgh and killed eleven Jewish Americans. When these kinds of crimes take place, it does not bode well for the host nation. Fortunately, President Trump has spoken out against the hate that inspired this massacre with great conviction. But President's Trump's declared support for a two-state solution in Israel made this possible. Interestingly, three days after Trump announced his support the gunman who attacked the synagogue posted pictures of all his guns on a site called Gab which is similar to Twitter.[xi] I'm not against posting pictures of one's guns but the fantasy of this shooter may have started developing after Trump's announcement. I believe President Trump's declaration opened a door into America that made it possible for Jews to be hated and attacked. I know without a doubt this was not his intention, but many empires and persons have been destroyed because they mistreated Israel and were unaware of the consequences it would bring. Anyways any nation that decides it will divide Israel will be judged and not prosper!

I will also gather all nations and bring them down to the Valley of Jehoshaphat; and I will enter into judgement with them there on account of My people, My heritage Israel, whom they have scattered among the nations; they have also divided up My land.

Joel 3:2 NKJV

The economy is not the only thing to be affected in America. Many prophets foresaw a red wave or Republican sweep in the midterms of 2018. I believe these prophets were not completely off the mark, but it was conditional on how they treated Israel. President Trump did well by retaining the U.S. Senate, but he could've won the House as well. He didn't win the House and now America is very divided because he supported a two-state solution on Israel and is presumably pushing such a policy behind the scene. He brought a curse of division upon America or replayed it again by supporting a two-state solution which previous administrations have done. President Trump needs to change this policy or his MAGA agenda will not succeed. I believe Jesus Christ wants America to be great, but unless Trump repents America will become very divided and the economy will be shaken greatly!

Anyone familiar with the stock market or the economy will understand there are two camps. There are the bulls and the bears. When the economy appears to be improving or is in a good state the bulls generally have the most influence. When the economy appears to be stagnant or failing the bears garner more influence. Like a person with bipolar disorder the market generally has extreme mood swings. One moment the bulls are charging ahead, and they believe the good times will never end, but on the other hand the bears could come out with a negative financial report and be terrorizing the market with fears of an inevitable collapse or depression. I believe that the python spirit can influence not only the mood of an individual, but a city or country.

But when her masters saw that their hope of profit was gone, they seized Paul and Silas and dragged them into the marketplace to the authorities. And they brought them to the magistrates, and said, "These men, being Jews, exceedingly trouble our city; and they teach customs which are not lawful for us being Romans, to receive or observe." Then the multitude rose up together against them; and the magistrates tore off their clothes and commanded them to be beaten with rods.

Acts 16:19-22 NKJV

Like the hysteria that took place in Paul's day the stock market can surge or plummet by the power of suggestion. The crowds or masses of investors can be easily compelled to buy or sell. This is done through famous personalities that speak on business news networks. One personality may say the debt of the U.S. cannot be fixed and that a financial collapse is imminent. They may suggest that people sell their stocks and invest in more tangible assets like gold. On the other hand, another analyst of the markets may suggest the exact opposite and encourage investors to buy stocks with the suggestion that the market will keep growing. Both opinions are an extreme and meant to keep investors in a constant state of uncertainty. Just as the python spirit sought to draw the crowds to Paul and Silas in order to manipulate the move of God these mouthpieces of the python spirit manipulate the masses today. A Christian should be careful when investing in the stock market for it is manipulated a great deal by the python spirit and other spirits. I believe intercessors and churches need to battle by prayer to see God the Father's kingdom come to the stock markets so that all the manipulation and fear controlling it can be broken. Until this takes place the markets of nations will go from bubbles to bubbles bursting and back to bubbles so that the finances of individuals are destroyed. This yoyo activity on the stock market could also destroy the finances of a nation and lead to devastating outcomes like revolution or war as we saw with World War 2! The roaring 20's was great, but so was the fall and the Great Depression which preceded World War 2.

Just as there are those who comment on the day to day trading and trends of the stock market there are those who report on the daily news. Cable news networks and blogs dedicated to the news are a phenomenon of our times, however, remember that python likes to control money and it has used money to control how the news is reported. There used to be a time when journalists and news organizations were more autonomous and concerned about real news, but this has changed as corporations bought up newspapers and news networks. Now this once noble profession has been corrupted by money and news organizations have essentially become instruments for propaganda. This is most evident in the United States where President Trump has managed to produce an economic miracle for the most part in America and for minorities who rarely see any change in their living standards. But you would think this economic miracle was not happening because President Trump is continually attacked in the media. The reason for this is that most news organizations are run by Democrats or globalists who are not too happy about Trump's America First policy. Even though the American Dream is being rebirthed in America these news organizations would have you believe we are in an American Nightmare! The python spirit loves to control the flow of information and the news. But you will rarely see these things anymore as the python spirit is using the media to constantly attack President Trump and make people believe things are horrible. Many are concerned that America has become very divided and see the media as the main culprit behind this division. Many now refer to the mainstream media as FAKE NEWS and have boycotted them. Fortunately, a freedom loving alternative media have sprung up to accommodate the angry and dissatisfied masses who have become disillusioned with mainstream news sources. But nearly half the U.S. still believe the lies of the mainstream media and that's enough to start a civil war. A house divided cannot stand and the python spirit knows this. It works tirelessly to convince the people through its liberal media empire that President Trump is evil incarnate. These deceived masses are deluded by this propaganda because this spirit has put a spell on them. They are unable to recognize the economic miracle taking place or any of the good news happening such as progress on talks with North Korea and their possible nuclear disarmament. When a people are under a spell or bewitched, they cannot think clearly despite the facts that are present.

O foolish Galatians! Who has bewitched you that you should not obey the truth, before whose eyes Jesus Christ was clearly portrayed among you as crucified?

Galatians 3:1 NKJV

Spiritual warfare must be employed against the python spirit so his grip on the news can be broken. The python spirit is only allowing people to see and hear bad news. These people are cursing their blessings without knowing it by proclaiming the bad news being given by the python spirit. Like Paul and Silas these people are sitting in a prison of their own making and thoughts. They must break free or be set free through the prayers and praise of the saints of the Most High God!

Python's Use of Hate, Fear and Intoxicants to Create Mob Violence

The spirit of python is a lawless spirit and it will attempt to rule any place it can with mob rule. When this spirit is not bound, and people have less respect for authority or any strong difference of opinion this spirit will hold sway over that area. In the city of Philippi, we see how the python spirit uses hate and fear to incite a riot.

When her owners realized that their hope of making money was gone, they seized Paul and Silas and dragged them into the marketplace to face the authorities. They brought them before the magistrates and said, "These men are Jews, and are throwing our city into an uproar by advocating customs unlawful for us Romans to accept or practice." The crowd joined in the attack against Paul and Silas, and the magistrates ordered them to be stripped and beaten with rods.

Acts 16:19-22 NIV

I don't know if there was a legal process through which damages could be claimed or the equivalent of a police force in Philippi, but if there were these slave masters ignored these routes. They essentially arrested Paul and Silas and forcefully brought them before the magistrates. The slave masters were angry because their slave girl could no longer divine after the python spirit was cast out by Paul in Jesus name. These slave masters pointed out to the magistrates that Paul and Silas were Jews and that they were teaching foreign beliefs. This angered the crowd for they feared that Paul and Silas represented a subversive element in their city. This xenophobia inspired the hate of the crowd without knowing anything about the case.

People can be manipulated/inspired to hate by the python spirit when it uses propaganda through its media mouthpieces. This hate can lead to violence and vigilante justice. In the case of Paul and Silas they were arrested by the slave masters who decided they were the law of the land.

There is one place in the U.S. where this mob violence is in operation and that is San Francisco. San Francisco like Philippi is a stronghold for ungodly customs. This city celebrates homosexuality, paganism and an assortment of other ungodly practices. Even though freedom of speech exists throughout the United States of America those controlled by the python spirit will stir up the people at places like Berkley University to hate any conservative guest speaker. Threats of violence and real violence are used to intimidate the speakers into not speaking at their event. If their threats fail to intimidate these speakers, their opponents will increase their threats and acts of violence until public safety seems seriously endangered. It is at this point Berkley University and the police will cancel the speaking engagement because they become concerned for the speaker's safety or the risk of a riot.[xii]

The python spirit will use political correctness, fear and unrighteous indignation to manipulate a people or government into silencing any voice of Conservatism or Christianity. This is illegal, but it is allowed to continue in the name of political correctness which is really a tool to censor anyone speaking about Jesus Christ or Conservative values.

The python spirit can really go into overdrive and create riots through the use of drugs, alcohol and propaganda. San Francisco and Berkley University weren't always hostile to Christian beliefs or Conservative values. The roots of this hostility were created through the rebellious period of 1960's San Francisco when a false peace was promoted. In the summer of 1967 many poured into San Francisco to have sex outside marriage (free love), do drugs and explore various occult ideas and psychology in an effort to escape the social conventions of the time.[xiii] They wanted a world without Jesus Christ and morality and got their wish for a time. During this time everyone celebrated peace and wanted nothing to do with an unpopular war in Viet Nam. Unfortunately, these people were not at peace, but at war with God. They wanted other religions, drugs and any kind of sex they wanted. This seed of rebellion would grow overtime and manifest once again in the homosexual culture for which San Francisco has became famous. San Francisco has been dubbed the "gay capital of the world."[xiv]

In a similar way, Sodom and Gommorah and the surrounding towns gave themselves up to sexual immorality and perversion. They serve as an example of those who suffer the punishment of eternal fire. In the very same way, on the strength of their dreams these ungodly people pollute their own bodies, reject authority and heap abuse on celestial beings.

Jude 1:7-8 NIV

Homosexuality did not develop in San Francisco because of love and rainbows, but due to hard hearts full of rebellion. The python spirit is a lawless spirit and will make a place devolve into anarchy. Jude wrote of a people who dream of ungodly things and a world without God. He mentions that they reject authority. The people who have gathered in San Francisco over the years have dreamed about a utopian world without God. These dreamers have minds which are influenced by drugs, alcohol and the New Age. This culture goes back to 1967 and continues today. The city of San Francisco could erupt at any moment like the city of Philippi if any controversial speaker visits their city. This culture of San Francisco has spread around the world to many cities. Like San Francisco these cities are ready to boil over and explode!

At this time, I'd like to comment on the rise of violent groups which are promoting and carrying out mob violence in American cities today. There are groups like ANTIFA and Proud Boys who are not afraid to engage violence and brawl on the streets. There is no doubt an influence of drugs and alcohol on the minds of these people.

ANTIFA has no real leader but consists of many loosely affiliated leftist groups some of whom will support everything from homosexuality and transgenderism to feminism and Communism. They identify themselves as a people who are against fascism and will use violence if necessary, to defeat those they deem to be fascists. They are often seen trying to intimidate Trump supporters and will attack them. They undoubtedly see President Trump as a fascist and therefore view his supporters as fascists.[xv] They fear their freedoms to practice their sexual sin, and other beliefs will be compromised by a President Trump. These violent protestors cannot see they are fascists themselves as they use violence to intimidate and harm those who support President Trump or other Conservative causes. Python controls ANTIFA through fear and encourages them to engage in lawless behaviour. These people are not being personally threatened for their lifestyle choices but are full of fear and fighting an imaginary enemy that they imagine Trump supporters to be. It is true there are Neo-Nazi groups in America, but Trump supporters are not haters and shouldn't be confused with Neo-Nazis. Python has used fear effectively and mobilized ANTIFA to increase lawlessness and persecute both Trump supporters and Christian believers.

Proud Boys was a group founded by Gavin McInnes. This man founded the group to defend against the erosion of Western Civilization and to restore the patriarchy.[xvi] When I look at some of their tenets I am in agreement, but I am concerned these guys are confusing drinking and tattoos with manhood. In addition, they believe one of the best ways they can prove their manhood and restore Western Civilization is through beating up Communists or members of ANTIFA. Western Civilization won't be restored through violence of the natural kind. It is only through spiritual warfare this can be achieved.

Finally, be strong in the Lord and in his mighty power. Put on the full armor of God, so that you can take your stand against the devil's schemes. For our struggle is not against flesh and blood, but against the rulers, against the authorities, against the powers of this dark world and against the spiritual forces of evil in heavenly realms.

Ephesians 6:10-12 NIV

As we can see from Ephesians 6 throwing punches will not change Western Civilization but overthrowing the spiritual rulers will. The python spirit knows there are people who long for a more traditional world and will manipulate them into thinking violence will change things. All violence will result in is increasing lawlessness and a cry from the people for order. Since python is a controlling spirit it will gladly add people to the prisons and bring martial law through the human rulers it controls. Violence is criminal behavior and won't lead to freedom. It will lead to a prison cell.

As people grow increasingly discontent with the way their country and the world are going, they will more likely become involved in some kind of faction or protest. These protests often involve alcohol and drugs. People often do reckless and violent acts when under the influence of alcohol and drugs. These substances give the python greater control over the people and they become vulnerable to the power of suggestion he whispers to their minds or through the megaphone of one of his speakers.

People have been manipulated into joining Crusades, Jihads, wars, riots and various social movements for centuries that often have nothing to do with God. These massive movements and wars are about fighting other human beings and not the real enemy. We don't need more armies with guns, but an army of prayer warriors!

The prayer of a righteous person is powerful and effective. Elijah was a human being, even as we are. He prayed earnestly that it would not rain, and it did

not rain on the land for three and a half years. Again he prayed, and the heavens gave rain, and the earth produced its crops.

James 5:16b-18 NIV

We need a prayer movement that would rally many Christians to town and city squares. We need prayer rallies in Washington D.C., New York City, Toronto, Paris, London, Rio de Janeiro, Delhi, Beijing, Johannesburg, Moscow, Tokyo and other cities around the world! We need not only prayers, but prayers coming from righteous people! Many are baffled why so many prayers are often having little effect. It is an issue of sin and the need for righteousness. When Christians begin to love righteousness as much as sinners love sin, they will shake heaven and earth with their prayers like Elijah!

The Python Spirit and its Religion of Rebellion

For rebellion is like the sin of divination, and arrogance like the evil of idolatry.

1 Samuel 15:23a NIV

The python spirit's religion of rebellion/witchcraft is perfectly on display in the United States of America. I hardly use Netflix anymore, but when I visit it there are a plethora of movies that are witchcraft based. Witchcraft has become the craze in America as it tries to throw off the shackles of Christianity. The influence of Christianity in an area restrains witchcraft, but only if it composed of obedient Christians. Many Christians are practising witchcraft without knowing it. The sin of rebellion is like divination or witchcraft and many Christians do not obey Jesus Christ or His word.

This religion started in the very beginning and gives us clues as to how it continues today. The first act of rebellion began with the woman in the Garden of Eden.

Now the serpent was more cunning than any beast of the field which the Lord God had made. And he said to the woman, "Has God indeed said, 'You shall not eat of every tree of the garden'?" And the woman said to the serpent, "We may eat the fruit of the trees of the garden; but of the fruit of the tree which is in the midst of the garden, God has said, 'You shall not eat it, nor shall you touch it, lest you die.'" Then the

serpent said to the woman, "You will not surely die. For God knows that in the day you eat of it your eyes will be opened, and you will be like God, knowing good and evil." So when the woman saw that the tree was good for food, that it was pleasant to the eyes, and a tree desirable to make one wise, she took of its fruit and ate. She also gave to her husband with her, and he ate. Then the eyes of both of them were opened, and they knew that they were naked; and they sewed fig leaves together and made themselves coverings.

Genesis 3:1-7 NKJV

In the beginning Eve rebelled against both God and Adam. The command to not eat of the tree of knowledge of good and evil was ignored. Rather than seek out Adam and consult with him she chose to instead in self-will to eat of the tree. She listened to the serpent's voice and not their voice. By doing so Eve aligned herself with God's archenemy Satan and a rebellious kingdom. Eve was never created to make unilateral decisions on major matters alone, but to be a helper to Adam (Genesis 2:18). This decision introduced a division between herself and Adam, however, she not only rebelled against Adam but also lead him into sin by offering him some of the fruit! Adam succumbed to Eve's suggestion and leadership and foolishly ate of the fruit. Many men do the same thing today and allow their wife or mother to lead them. Rather than engage in an uncomfortable confrontation with the woman about her manipulation he avoids the issue and hides away. Fortunately, God set something in place to prevent the rebellion and manipulation of the woman from ever totally eclipsing the authority of the man.

To the woman He said: "I will greatly multiply your sorrow and conception; in pain you shall bring forth children; your desire shall be for your husband, and he shall rule over you." Then to Adam He said, "Because you have heeded the voice of your wife, and have eaten from the tree of which I commanded you, saying, 'You shall not eat of it': "Cursed is the ground for your sake; in toil you shall eat of it all the days of your life. Both thorns and thistles it shall bring forth for you, and you shall eat the herb of the field. In the sweat of your face you shall eat bread till you return to the ground, for out of it you were taken; for dust you are, and to dust you shall return."

Genesis 3:16-19 NKJV

In these verses we can see that the woman's desire for her husband or her attempt to lead him as Eve originally did would continue, but the man would rule over her. As a consequence of Adam lazily agreeing to eat the fruit at Eve's suggestion Adam and men through all time would constantly work and fight the resistance of the earth when thorns and thistles would grow up. Adam and men would be constantly fighting to rule their women and the land.

When men rule society it is not perfect, but it generally follows the pattern set by God. Unfortunately, men do not always rule like they are supposed to and let women lead them. This leads to disaster and the result is the destruction of family, nations and civilizations! Through Eve all of mankind was introduced to the destructive consequences of sin and she disqualified herself from being a leader. Some believe men and women can rule together, but this is not possible. God ordained the man to rule the woman and she would be his helper. Just as sin entered the world through Eve it has entered the world through the woman once again and leading us into a great apostasy. This has never happened before because the woman has generally played a subordinate role to man over the centuries, but this changed in the 20th century. Like Adam men failed to rule over the woman and instead allowed themselves to be led by women once again. As a result, the religion of rebellion/witchcraft was introduced into America and Western Civilization. I will now unveil this religion that the python spirit rules over and how it has manifested over time.

To simplify things, I will give this religion a name that is already in use today. This religion of python which manifests in rebellion and divination can be better understood as Communism. Communism seeks to overthrow any hierarchy that it deems oppressive. At the end of the day Communism hates all forms of authority and will keep inventing new classes of people who are oppressed. According to Facebook there are 50-71 gender options![xvii] Can you see what happens when we reject God's order of things and adapt a Babylonian system of understanding? Babylon means "confusion" and outside of God's law that's all there is. Rebellion or wickedness always leads to chaos and a lack of peace. Those who follow Communism or the python spirit's ways of rebellion will never experience peace!

Go forth from Babylon! Flee from the Chaldeans! With a voice of singing, Declare, proclaim this, utter it to the end of the earth; say, "The Lord has redeemed His servant Jacob!" And they did not thirst when He led them through the deserts; He caused the waters to flow from the rock for them; He also split the rock, and the waters gushed out. "There is no peace," says the Lord, "for the wicked."

Isaiah 48:20-22 NKJV

I find it interesting that while the Russian Revolution took place in Russia during the year 1917 the woman's right to vote came into power in 1920 in the United States. These events both happened in the 20th century. When God created the earth, we saw a division happen between light and darkness. He also divided the water and the sky on the second day of creation. For this reason, the number 2 represents division. Therefore, the woman's right to vote being made legal in 1920 in the 20th century represents a time of division and the rebellion of the woman to man's authority. The woman's right to vote and Communism were an attack on legitimate authority set up by God and He approved of neither. Both feminism and Communism work together very closely to overthrow the patriarchy and God's rule in America and throughout the earth. Is it any wonder they do so when they were birthed at the same time? The Russian Revolution removed the tsar of Russia and ended the monarchy of Russia. In the United States the 19th Amendment gave women the right to vote, but in reality, it was the woman asserting she was equal with the man in authority. The idea being asserted here is that the woman is an oppressed class and needed to be liberated from the man. We just saw an election take place on November 6, 2018 in the U.S. midterms and it revealed the deep divide and rebellion in America. A hated President Trump represents the white male patriarchy that defends tradition and Christianity and a white female Nancy Pelosi representing the matriarchy ruling the House of Representatives. Some may argue that it doesn't matter that she's a woman, but only her beliefs. That is a lie and God will not tolerate this lie any longer. He wants men to lead again and for women to submit to male authority! I will now quote verses which clearly limit the role of the woman and her need to defer to the authority of the man in case you think I'm a misogynistic woman hater. I do not hate women, but there is a clear line of authority from God!

As for My people, children are their oppressors, and woman rule over them. O My people! Those who lead you cause you to err, and destroy the way of your paths."

Isaiah 3:12 NKJV

Take note that when women and children rule a people they will be led into error and be destroyed!

And I do not permit a woman to teach or to have authority over a man, but to be in silence. For Adam was formed first, then Eve. And Adam was not deceived, but the woman being deceived, fell into transgression. Nevertheless she will be saved in childbearing if they continue in faith, love, and holiness, with self-control. This is a faithful saying: <u>If a man</u> desires the position of a bishop, he desires a good work. A bishop then must be blameless, <u>the husband of one wife</u>, temperate, sober-minded, of good behavior, hospitable, able to teach;

1 Timothy 2:12-3:1-2 NKJV

Any women reading the above text must submit to God and step down from any teaching position or pastoral role where they are leading men. God called only men to guide the Church from the pulpit and the men allowing women to be pastors must repent and stop being spineless jellyfish! God called you men to rule over the women, but many of you have failed to do that and as a result the woman is ruling for the most part because you abdicated your role as King Ahab did when he succumbed to his wife Jezebel. Now the spirit of Jezebel along with the python spirit run rampant in society and in the Church. We no longer have a patriarchy, but a matriarchy. Fortunately, God is raising up men like President Trump, President Putin and Jair Bolsonaro (President-elect of Brazil) to teach men how to lead again and without apology! It must be stated that men must not only rule the woman but do it in love. Men must be firm but loving.

Husbands, love your wives, just as Christ also loved the church and gave Himself for her,

Ephesians 5:25 NKJV

Unfortunately, men did not rule the women as they should have before women protested and demanded the right to vote. Women were at times reduced to a slave and not allowed to have any dreams or ambitions of their own. God never wanted the woman to be chained up in a kitchen, but He did want her to submit to the authority of the man. According to Proverbs 31 women can operate their own businesses and are encouraged to do so. In addition, we know that Miriam and Deborah were prophets. I believe women can do almost anything, but they are restricted from holding executive positions of authority or power such as a pastor, police officer, soldier or politician. Anyone who disagrees with that is likely living in rebellion or has been brainwashed by popular culture. Many want to see abortion and gay marriage defeated, but do not recognize that the root sin of female rebellion or feminism is what empowers these abominations and made them possible. In fact, before women gained the right to vote in 1920 Margaret Sanger the founder of Planned Parenthood opened the first birth control clinic in the United States in the year 1916 for which she was arrested. Therefore, any victory over abortion will only be achieved when men lead again, and women yield to male authority again. Abortion would never had become a reality if women continued to obey their husbands and not insisted on voting. But men relinquished their authority to rule the woman again and we saw abortion become legalized later on in 1973 in the name of women's rights.

When I was writing earlier on in this chapter you likely remember me mentioning that President Trump represents a white male patriarchy. When I wrote this, I did not intend to be offensive, but in reality, it is true. In every nation there will usually be dominant racial group. Anyone travelling to any nation will quickly find out who is the dominant racial group. No racial group should have to apologize for their dominant position if their population is the largest, but neither should they look down on other races as inferior. Every nation needs a common language, culture and a dominant racial group. Multiculturalism will never succeed, and it is only a tool to destroy white people who have a Christian heritage. Whites and minorities have been taught that white people are responsible for most evil in the world and that they are oppressing others economically. Whites are not oppressing anyone, but they are the majority and naturally will hold most influential positions or jobs. Unfortunately, this has changed, and minorities are being taught that they are entitled to have everything white people have. As a result, the government and corporations are ensuring that minorities are having access and control of jobs that whites traditionally held. It is for this reason some will never accept a President Trump because he is a white male person and they want a post-White America. This agenda is rebellious towards the majority racial group and an attempt to overthrow them. The false teachings empowering this agenda will only create division and rebellion. Immigrants and minorities should expect to be treated with decency and protest any genuine mistreatment, but to plot the overthrow of white people is manipulation and not of God.

The cultural Marxism we see today is a tactic of the python spirit to carry out its rebellious agenda and turn people against one another. We all have to submit to someone in life and we can't blame others for our position in life. We are not all equal in position, wealth, talent or opportunity. But we can change these things through hard work. Being a victim will never change one's status but working hard toward a goal will. We must be realistic about what we can achieve or what we are entitled to. If we refuse to do this, we will see the fruits of rebellion or divination and live in a very divided country or world.

But Jesus knew their thoughts, and said to them: "Every kingdom divided against itself is brought to desolation, and every city or house divided against itself will not stand.

Matthew 12:25 NKJV

The Python Spirit's Role in Mental Illness, Sicknesses, Drug Addiction, Prisons and Medicine

In the 16th chapter of the book of Acts we were introduced to the spirit of python and discovered that his ultimate goal is the enslavement of a person. We have discussed some of the ways he has done this, but we only talked about mental illness and drug addiction a bit. These two issues can no longer be put off by this book or society. They must be addressed and dealt with!

The governments of our day do not want to deal with the massive expenditure of treating mental illness and the already costly war on drugs in the U.S. seems to never end. It is my belief that these twin issues will never be solved until we deal with our rebellion towards God. In the previous chapter we examined how the python spirit rules over a religion of rebellion. That may have seemed simplistic to some, but it is the truth. Most doctors want to convince us that every malady under the sun is a chemical imbalance and that it can be corrected with a pill. This is rebellion as we are trying to address the problem without God and godlessness is the reason for why we have so many drug addicts and mentally ill people suffering around us today. Our rebellion towards God has brought this upon us.

"But it shall come to pass, if you do not obey the voice of the Lord your God, to observe carefully all His commandments and His statutes which I command you today, that all these curses will come upon you and overtake you: "The Lord will cause you to be defeated before your enemies; you shall go out one way against them and flee seven ways before them; and you shall be troublesome to all the kingdoms of the earth. The Lord will strike you with the boils of Egypt, with tumors, with the scab, and with the itch, <u>from which you cannot be healed</u>. The Lord will strike you with madness and blindness and confusion of heart.

Deuteronomy 28:15, 25, 27-28 NKJV

Let me state clearly that I am not against medications for the treatment of mental illness or medications that treat other illnesses. But it is my belief that we have ignored the root cause for most of our illnesses which is rebellion towards God's commands. Many people take medications to manage their moods or health conditions. But have you ever noticed that these medications never heal the illness, but only manage the symptoms? Take note that in the 27th verse I posted above it states there are illnesses which cannot be healed. In particular, tumors are mentioned as being one of the diseases which cannot be healed. I believe this is referring to cancer which is one of the deadliest diseases one can acquire.

I believe that Jesus Christ can work through modern medicine to bring about something close to a cure for cancer or at least a way to manage it. Cancer can be a stubborn disease to remove because most people are receiving treatment through medicine alone. Doctors are using radiation, surgery, medications and other methods to remove cancer. The radiation treatment can damage the immune system and cause many other illnesses. These treatments are crude, but they do keep people alive longer. Sometimes people are fortunate enough to see their cancer go into remission after treatment, but it can and often does make a comeback. The reason for this is that cancer is incurable apart from God as we read in Deuteronomy. I'm certain that most cases where cancer goes into permanent remission is a result of prayer. Many have turned to Jesus Christ when facing this illness and find some healing. In some cases, people are completely healed by Jesus Christ. Cancer is a demon and it must be cast out in Jesus name. Apart from Jesus Christ true healing for cancer is unattainable. The python spirit wants the cancer patient to trust in the magic of medicine alone and will at times permit a recovery to convince the patient they "need" medications to stay in such a state of recovery. This results in the patient taking medication for the rest of their lives and having a constant dependence on some kind of pill (s). In other words, the patient becomes a slave to the medication and Big Pharma which is ruled over by the python spirit.

Like cancer there are many other illnesses that cannot be healed, but only managed with medicine. In the passage above I quoted from Deuteronomy it mentions some of the curses that come as a result of disobedience. They are defeat, fleeing, madness and confusion of heart. These symptoms sound very much like mental illness. The python spirit can cause many of these problems. When we looked at the python spirit's operation in the city of Philippi in the second chapter, we discovered that the jailer overseeing the imprisonment of Paul and Silas was depressed and suicidal. Most of the city of Philippi was populated by slaves and this jailer was part of this system. One cannot oppress and control others through slavery or manipulation and expect to be immune to the crushing hopelessness of the python spirit!

We already looked at how python rules over a rebellious system. Many people break the law because this spirit of python drives them to disobey any and all authority. This results in their imprisonment and once they get out, they often become repeat offenders. This spirit gives their host the impression that their criminal life is an indication they are free from all constraints and independent. But they are deceived and unaware that rebellion leads to slavery or captivity. Some crimes can lead to imprisonment for life. The criminal thinks they can manage their criminal behavior so that they are not committing the most serious offenses and get out later. But association with crime will eventually lead to more serious crimes because the criminal does not realize they have already lost control. It is ironic that the nation that loves freedom so much is in reality a nation of slaves. I am referring to the U.S. and its sky-high prison population.[xviii] Many Americans confuse freedom with lawlessness, but freedom does not equate to lawlessness. True freedom can only be found in the love that Jesus Christ supplies.

There is no fear in love. But perfect love drives out fear, because fear has to do with punishment. The one who fears is not made perfect in love.

1 John 4:18 NIV

Those who love their fellow man will not harm them. But those who harm their fellow man will always be on the lookout in the fear their crime will be discovered. Some think that they are tough and that they can protect themselves through violence and intimidation. They are always in a state of survival, but never at rest. Fear is slavery, but love is freedom.

In the U.S. the problem with drug addiction has become an epidemic. This scourge of drug addiction is very much connected with the large number of people incarcerated. Most recreational drugs are illegal and as a result it usually requires some contact with criminals to acquire. Unfortunately, those addicted to drugs are enslaved to a slave master we would call a drug pusher today. At first the drug is used to manage some kind of emotional pain or simply for the pursuit of pleasure. The drug dealer is controlled by the python spirit like the drug addict. The drug addict imagines that what they are participating in is not criminal and that they are not a criminal like the drug pusher. But the drug addict eventually finds out their drug addiction is unsustainable for they need more and more of the drug. This habit will become unaffordable at some point and the drug pusher is not charitable in any way. When the addict cries out to the drug pusher for a fix that they cannot afford their cries will be ignored. A shocking revelation comes to the drug addict that he/she needs help or that they will have to become a criminal like the drug pusher in order to continue their addiction. Many do not find the help they need and begin their new life as a criminal. Eventually the drug addict gets caught by the police and put in jail. Many are in jail because of an addiction. The Lord Jesus Christ wants to free the many slaves of the python spirit who dwell in prison. I believe there is coming great freedom to many drug addicts, criminals and those who maintain this prison system. The python spirit wants us to believe that criminals cannot be reformed and that the cold prison system cannot change, but Jesus Christ says otherwise. I have a prophecy I'd like to share at this point.

I prophesy by faith in the name of Jesus Christ that a great emancipation is coming to the prisoners of the python spirit in these last days! These prisoners of

hope will be overflowing with the joy of the Lord and the love of Jesus Christ. The prisons will no longer overflow with sin, but grace! Prisoners will be truly reformed by the power and grace of God. These former places of hopelessness will become places of revival! God wants a prayer movement to start in the prisons so that He can come in power and shake off the chains of sin and break the power of the python spirit. Can I not redeem those who have murdered like I redeemed David, Moses and Paul? Do not give up hope for these prisoners of hope for I desire to break the power of hopelessness that is ruling from these prisons. I am planning a prison break through an outbreak of hope in the hearts of these hopeless ones and the prison doors will be opened!

The Spirit of the Sovereign Lord is on me, because the Lord has anointed me to proclaim good news to the poor. He has sent me to bind up the brokenhearted, to proclaim freedom for the captives and release from darkness for the prisoners, to proclaim the year of the Lord's favor and the day of vengeance of our God, to comfort all who mourn, and provide for those who grieve in Zion—to bestow on them a crown of beauty instead of ashes, the oil of joy instead of mourning, and a garment of praise instead of a spirit of despair. They will be called oaks of righteousness, a planting of the Lord for the display of his splendor.

Isaiah 61:1-3 NIV

Fortunately, most people that are oppressed by the python spirit do not dwell in physical prisons. But many are imprisoned in the spiritual prisons of python. Many of those with mental illnesses, sicknesses and drug addictions have been told the lie that a medication or drug can fix their situation. But these drugs never heal the people, but only give the illusion they are being healed or made better. These drugs only manage their symptoms, but their underlying condition is unchanged for the most part. Therefore, these prisoners of the python spirit continue to believe the lie that there is a magic pill out there that will fix their problem not realizing they have been deceived by sorcery.

The light of a lamp shall not shine in you anymore, and the voice of the bridegroom and bride shall not be heard in you anymore. For your merchants were the great men of the earth, for by your sorcery all the nations were deceived.

Revelation 18:23 NKJV

In the above verse the translators used the word "sorcery" to best represent what was being spoken in the Greek. The Greek word for sorcery is transliterated as "pharmakeia" from which we get the word pharmacy! This industry has made people believe medicine is the answer to all illnesses, but it is all a lie to stop us from seeking out Jesus Christ for healing. I'm not saying Jesus Christ can't use some medications to help us cope or deal with something like an infection nor am I saying we should stop taking any prescribed medications. My point is that this system is teaching us we don't need Jesus Christ and that the best we can hope for is to manage our symptoms or sicknesses.

At the beginning of the book I mentioned the myth of the python and how it was killed by the Greek god Apollo. Both python and Apollo were known for their prophetic abilities. Apollo was not only known for his prophetic abilities, but his healing ability as well. Interestingly a serpent is connected with modern day medicine via a symbol that is also connected with the son of Apollo who was named Asclepius.[xix]

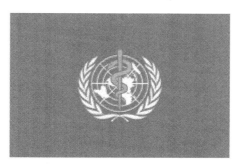

I have posted a picture of this symbol used by the U.N.'s World Health Organization. Have no doubt this spirit of python or Apollo have worldwide influence over the practice of medicine. This ancient serpent was connected with destruction[xx], but still used as a symbol of healing. Guess what? The name Apollo means "Destroyer".[xxi] I am convinced these three commonalities of python and Apollo make them one and the same. Both are connected with prophecy, healing and associated with destruction. Hmmm isn't there a character in the Bible by this name?

They had as king over them the angel of the Abyss, whose name in Hebrew is Abaddon and in Greek is Apollyon (that is, Destroyer).

Revelation 9:11 NIV

If you have any doubt about Apollo's connection to medicine or his connection to Asclepius let me post here the oath the majority of physicians take when becoming a doctor. This oath was created by one who is considered to be the father of medicine in the Western world. His name was Hippocrates.

I swear by <u>Apollo</u> the Healer, by <u>Asclepius</u>, by <u>Hygieia</u>, by <u>Panacea</u>, and by all the gods and goddesses, making them my witnesses, that I will carry out, according to my ability and judgment, this oath and this indenture.

To hold my teacher in this art equal to my own parents; to make him partner in my livelihood; when he is in need of <u>money to share</u> mine with him; to consider his family as my own brothers, and to teach them this art, if they want to learn it, without fee or indenture; to impart precept, oral instruction, and all other instruction to my own sons, the sons of my teacher, and to indentured pupils who have taken the physician's oath, but to nobody else.

I will use treatment to help the sick according to my ability and judgment, but never with a view to injury and wrong-doing. Neither will I administer a poison to anybody when asked to do so, nor will I suggest such a course. Similarly I will not give to a woman a <u>pessary</u> to cause abortion. But I will keep pure and holy both my life and my art. I will not use the knife, not even, verily, on sufferers from <u>stone</u>, but I will give place to such as are craftsmen therein.

Into whatsoever houses I enter, I will enter to help the sick, and I will abstain from all intentional wrong-doing and harm, especially from abusing the bodies of <u>man or woman</u>, <u>bond or free</u>. And whatsoever I shall see or hear in the course of my profession, as well as outside my profession in my intercourse with men, if it be what should not be published abroad, I will never divulge, holding such things to be holy secrets.

Now if I carry out this oath, and break it not, may I gain for ever reputation among all men for my life and for my art; but if I break it and forswear myself, may the opposite befall me.[4] - Translation by <u>James Loeb</u>.[xxii]

It gets even stranger because this python/Apollo spirit not only controls medicine, but diseases as well! One of his titles was "Apollo of the Plague".[xxiii] Actually, this spirit has great influence over New York City. In a later chapter we will look at how the python/Apollo spirit has its throne in New York City and rules from there!

Before we continue to the next chapter, I'd just like to say that this python/Apollo spirit likes to imprison people in a hopeless state. We saw how this spirit rules over the Abyss or hell which is a prison. This spirit also enslaved the people of Philippi and subjected Paul and Silas to imprisonment. This spirit claims to be a healer, but in reality, is a destroyer. It destroys people through drug addiction, medications that have numerous side effects and the lie that one does not need Jesus Christ to be healed and saved. This spirit loves to be the Word of God like Jesus Christ through false prophecy and a healer. But his real goal is our destruction in the Abyss and an eternity without Jesus Christ! If you do not know Jesus Christ as your Lord and Savior, I urge you to immediately repent of all your sins and stop trusting in the deception of medication aka sorcery alone. Invite Jesus Christ into your life. Jesus Christ wants to heal you completely body, soul and spirit and deliver you from an eternity in hell.

He sent out His word and healed them, and delivered them from their destructions.

Psalm 107:20 NKJV

Python's Use of False Prophecy and Witchcraft Today

Before I write about the explosion of the occult in the world today, I would first like to talk about false prophecy in the Church. I believe we are and will continue to see an increase of false prophecy in the Church as righteousness declines. In fact, it is already rampant in the Church because of one word which is largely absent from the lips of prophets and lay people today. The word I am referring to is "REPENT". I believe this is the main reason why many have fallen away, and it will accelerate us towards the appearance of the antichrist or lawless one. The lawless one will arrive because of the sin which will break out in many churches. There will also be a lack of teaching on or practise of repentance. Why then is there so little teaching or prophecy in regard to repentance these days?

Preach the word; be prepared in season and out of season; correct, rebuke and encourage—with great patience and careful instruction. For the time will come when people will not put up with sound doctrine. Instead, to suit their own desires, they will gather around them a great number of teachers to say what their itching ears want to hear. They will turn their ears away from the truth and turn aside to myths. But you, keep your head in all situations,

endure hardship, do the work of an evangelist, discharge all the duties of your ministry.

2 Timothy 4:2-5 NIV

<u>Myths</u>

Paul gives us several reasons for why there is little teaching or prophecy on repentance. One of the reasons is that people would rather hear about myths than the truth. We live in a culture where people love Hollywood movies! This is the reason why I spent little time at the beginning of the book talking about the myth of Python/Apollo because this spirit loves to tell stories or create myths all in an effort to lead people astray from the Bible. I totally believe in having encounters with angels sent by Jesus Christ and that there are times Jesus Christ could call us up to heaven like John in the Book of Revelation, but my concern is that some people claim to be constantly encountering angels and seeing heaven. Paul warned about such people in his letter to the church at Colossae (Colossians 2:18-19). They are always talking about some new revelation, but there is little evidence of the fear of the Lord in their lives. I believe the Lord Jesus Christ allows some of us to encounter various visions. Some of these visions will be true and others false. It is a test to see whether we truly love His word more than the spiritual experiences themselves. All spiritual experiences must be judged by the Bible. There are some books about angels and heaven that people are promoting to be on equal grounds with the Bible. Of course, they won't say that directly, but suggest it by other means. When this takes place, people start looking to books instead of the Bible.

It's Not Cool or It's Out of Season

The Church in the West has been constantly retreating on social values. The reason for this is that the Ahab spirit is controlling most men. Men were led to believe that women should be equal in authority and were reluctant to assert their authority when women started crying about how unfair things were. Women got their voting rights and here we are today. Did we progress closer to God? No, but we did see a great apostasy in the 60's because we opened a big door of rebellion through allowing women to vote. There is nothing unfair about authority it simply must be obeyed. Those who are not in power will always complain about how unfair things are, but they are just rebels who don't want to submit to the legitimate authority in power. Women and children will always rebel against the male who plays the role husband and father. He must rule them with a firm love and without apology. Rebels can always sense weakness and will persist until you show real strength. I've learned this by dealing with a number of people in my life.

Feminists are a rebellious faction that want to overthrow the patriarchy. I just found out the other day that patriarchy means "rule of the father". Feminists who have a Jezebel spirit will by no means abide by a patriarchal system because of their shared hate for God the Father. God purposely uses male pronouns when referring to Himself in the Bible. Whether it be the Father, Son or the Holy Spirit they are all referred to as "He". Paul mentioned that we need to preach the word in season and out of season. Instructing women to submit to their husbands and to relinquish their claim to the pulpit may not seem too modern, but its Biblical! I'm not trying to pick on women in this book, but I am trying to do my part to set things in order. The reason why we keep retreating on social issues is that men conceded their authority when they allowed women to vote and they won't be too powerful until they take it back and rule over the women. Like Adam they allowed Eve to lead and became complacent. This is why men must struggle through work because Adam took the easy way out and ate the fruit when he should've corrected Eve. As a result, the man will always face challenges to his rule from his wife and children because of Adam's neglect in being a leader! His life will be one of constant struggle.

Abortion came as a result of woman's rights. The homosexual and transgender lifestyles came about as the role of women and men became redefined as a result of a woman's right to vote. Women are behaving more like men and men more like women. I know some will disagree with my conclusions here, but anyone wanting to follow Jesus and the truth will hear me. The root of all these social problems is the rebellion of women and the abdication of men who surrendered their authority to appear modern. They wanted the world to love them.

The python spirit you will remember is essentially a spirit of rebellion. Samuel said rebellion is like the sin of divination. The python spirit will work to promote the idea of egalitarianism within and without the Church. It seems like a fair idea to many, but it is in rebellion to God's call on the man to lead. We have nothing close to an egalitarian system today, but we do have a matriarchal system which is presently being challenged by the rise of powerful male figures in government. Some examples are President Trump in the U.S., Vladimir Putin in Russia and the recent election of Jair Bolsonaro in Brazil. God the Father is establishing His kingdom on earth so we better line up with His agenda!

No Sound Doctrine and Itching Ears

There is a very popular teacher in the Charismatic church who purposely distorts the Scriptures to create a Jesus no one can fear. He says, "Jesus Christ is perfect theology." I agree that Jesus Christ is perfect theology, but this teacher claims Jesus Christ never causes anyone to become sick or kill them. This is a lie for he intentionally ignores what Jesus Christ said to the 7 churches of Revelation. In the message to these churches He said He would kill some, cause others to get sick unless they repented. This teacher wants a Jesus of his own making and not the Jesus Christ of Scripture. False teachers/prophets always take Scripture out of context by picking only one part that they like to follow or distorting the meaning. He proclaims God's goodness without any fear of the Lord. False teachers/prophets generally follow an extreme path for they typically over emphasize God's goodness or His role as Judge. This same Jesus who is loving will cast people into hell for eternity for rejecting and disobeying Him. Therefore, we must be balanced in how we perceive Jesus Christ by embracing all He has said in the Bible!

Therefore consider the goodness and severity of God: on those who fell, severity; but toward you, goodness, if you continue in His goodness. Otherwise you also will be cut off.

Romans 11:22 NKJV

It is at this point I want to expand on how the python spirit creates extremes in the prophetic. Usually people find themselves in either camp of the prophetic. When people only expose themselves to one style of the prophetic, they are in danger of falling into error and coming under the influence of the python spirit.

Our theology is very important for it determines the filter through which we prophesy. For example, if we believe God is perpetually kind and never judges, we are unlikely to hear or speak a prophetic rebuke. Some people confuse being positive with how God speaks. In their world anything that doesn't involve their personal happiness could not be from God. They selectively pick out the attributes of God they like and ignore those they dislike. But God isn't always concerned with our happiness, but the state of our souls. There may be sin that we need to repent of and He will rebuke or correct us. If there was a sin in your life which could lead you to hell wouldn't you want Him to point it out? You may object at this point and say you said a sinner's prayer. A sinner's prayer is a great way to begin our journey towards heaven. But salvation is not an event, but a walk! As we saw in the verse above it is about continuing in His goodness and not some magic formula. Even though we can receive correction through a prophecy the Lord Jesus is trying to encourage us the majority of the time. Therefore, we need to understand that Jesus Christ is not perpetually angry with us, but at times He can correct us.

But he who prophesies speaks edification and exhortation and comfort to men.

1 Corinthians 14:3 NKJV

One of the reasons I love Jesus Christ is that He is always encouraging me, and He typically will be doing the same with you. He never gives up on me and for that reason I never give up on the idea that any sin in my life can be defeated. Through Jesus Christ I can do all things! In the above verse I can see Jesus Christ is concerned with building us up, urging us forward in life and comforting us. But there are some who think Jesus Christ is constantly on a hunt to expose all our sins. Every prophecy or sermon delivered by these teachers/prophets leave us feeling unworthy or condemned. We don't feel inspired towards a goal or loved by God but condemned. When these preachers look at the world, they see it as hopelessly wicked and irredeemable. The only hope they offer is the rapture to deliver us from this dark world. But this is not how Jesus Christ sees the world. When He came into the world, He was the light of the world.

Then Jesus spoke to them again, saying, "I am the light of the world. He who follows Me shall not walk in darkness, but have the light of life."

John 8:12 NKJV

The world was a much darker place when Jesus Christ came and has become much better because of Him. Through His sacrifice on the cross He has redeemed us back to God the Father. His teachings revolutionized the way we think and are the basis of many of our laws. Unfortunately, many are not as aware of the teachings of Jesus Christ today. We are distracted by so many televisions shows, movies, cellphones, tablets and other things. It seems like we live in the darkest of times, but this is not a time to lament. When things are darkest that's when the best things of God show up! Most of the prophets we read about in the Bible came in the most trying of times. Moses appeared when Israel was in slavery for approximately 400 years and delivered them. Elijah came on the scene when the worship of God was nearly destroyed throughout Israel. He brought revival and destroyed Baal worship in Israel. We should not despair but be prepared to be used by God. Don't listen to the doom and gloom prophets who only see the darkness, but shine!

Arise, shine; for your light has come! And the glory of the Lord is risen upon you. For behold, the darkness shall cover the earth, and deep darkness the people; but the Lord will arise over you, and His glory will be seen upon you. The Gentiles shall come to your light, and kings to the brightness of your rising.

Isaiah 60:1-3 NKJV

The verses I posted above refer to the last days when spiritual darkness covers the earth. Fortunately, the darkness will not win, but only if we shine! Jesus Christ calls us to arise and shine and to stop wallowing in despair. The fight can be very intense, but through Jesus Christ we can do all things.

One of the ways we can detect false prophecy and false prophets is how they speak. They will usually speak with flattery to get your money or judge and curse you.

But there were also false prophets among the people, even as there will be false teachers among you, who will secretly bring in destructive heresies, even denying the Lord who bought them, and bring on themselves swift destruction. And many will follow their destructive ways, because of whom the way of truth will be blasphemed. By covetousness they will exploit you with deceptive words; for a long time their judgement has not been idle, and their destruction does not slumber.

2 Peter 2:1-3 NKJV

My brethren, let not many of you become teachers, knowing that we shall receive a stricter judgement. Out of the same mouth proceed blessing and cursing. My brethren, these things ought not to be so.

James 3:1, 10 NKJV

In conclusion, false prophets in the Church will follow some kind of extreme. Either they speak words which are only sweet (flattery) or only corrective words on a constant basis. In both extremes one either feels inflated with pride or completely unworthy. False prophets will not use the Bible much but rely more on their "revelations". True prophets on the other hand will have a balanced approach by bringing both encouragement and correction and use Scripture frequently.

Then the voice which I heard from heaven spoke to me again and said, "Go, take the little book which is open in the hand of the angel who stands on the sea and on the earth." So I went to the angel and said to him, "Give me the little book." And he said to me, "Take and eat it; and it will make your stomach bitter, but it will be as sweet as honey in your mouth." Then I took the little book out of the angel's hand and ate it, and it was as sweet as honey in my mouth. But when I had eaten it, my stomach became bitter. And he said to me, "You must prophesy again about many peoples, nations, tongues, and kings."

Revelation 10:8-11 NKJV

Witchcraft in the World Today

In North America and other areas of the world today we see a rising interest in witchcraft. It is not surprising that we are witnessing this as there is so much rebellion these days. Witchcraft presents itself as being new, but it is old like Christianity and the Bible. I will try my best to inform you on how you can best discern witchcraft in the world today. Witchcraft likes to appear instantaneous in nature. There is this idea that if one casts a spell all their problems will disappear. Nothing is free, and witchcraft will only lead to bondage.

Divination

The spirit of python/divination controls divination or the area of magic concerned with foresight or hidden knowledge. Witches will use tarot cards, Ouija boards, rune stones, astrology, palm reading and an assortment of other means to finding secret knowledge about people and the future. There are many ways to divine, but all these methods have one thing in common. These methods use objects or the stars to arrive at answers to the mysteries of life. They don't require any faith. Witches manipulate these objects through the power of a python spirit knowingly or unknowingly. In some cases, like the Oracle of Delphi or the slave girl with the python spirit in the book of Acts they will merely prophesy with their mouth. But these diviners will never confess Jesus Christ is Lord or lead others to Jesus Christ.

Sorcery or Casting Spells

Just as divination manipulates objects to discover secret knowledge those who practise sorcery manipulate energy in order to empower their spells. But the energy they feel, and use is the power of the python spirit. Sorcery is employed to manipulate people, events and places in favor of one's own desires. Basically, the witch is playing god and making things happen. They are not waiting on God for an answer but are using witchcraft to impose their will on people, events and places. We must be careful to pray God's will for people and not our own will. To impose our will upon others through prayer is no different than what a sorcerer does. It is manipulation and we must never confuse manipulation with faith. Manipulation is trust in our own ability, but faith is trust in God's ability.

Meditation, Yoga, Martial Arts and Astral Travel

Meditation, yoga, martial arts and astral travel are about manipulating a person's own body through occult power. They involve assuming a certain pose or posture to achieve a spiritual state. In the case of martial arts, one is being empowered by demons to achieve unnatural results like breaking boards and bricks. With astral travel a person relaxes to such a point where they feel they can leave their body and travel with their spiritual body.

Superstition

Whether it be a rabbit's foot or some kind of ritual supposed to bring luck these things are all about trusting in something other than Jesus Christ. Many Christians are involved in superstition when they wear a cross in the hope it brings safety. Safety is not found in crosses around our necks, but rebuking evil in the name of Jesus Christ! We trust in Jesus Christ and not in superstitious activities or items.

Gods and Idols

Yes, people do worship false gods today. In the religion of Hinduism there are many gods and goddesses. In Roman Catholicism people essentially make Mary the mother of Jesus a goddess. They pray the rosary and trust in Mary. There is no place in the Bible where we are instructed to worship or pray to Mary. In addition, Catholics will pray to saints and angels like they are gods who they believe to oversee certain areas of life. Before Christianity there were many gods in the mythology of different nations that were believed to rule over certain areas of life. The Egyptians, Babylonians, Greeks and Romans had their pantheon of gods and goddesses in their mythology. There are witches who worship or pray to these false gods today and idols that supposedly look like them.

Spirit Guides

Spirit guides are a spirit that New Agers call upon to guide them. They are counterfeiters of the Holy Spirit. The python spirit and other spirits carry out this function to get people dependant on them and not God. Sometimes these spirits are called a familiar spirit in the Bible. These spirits know us well for they are "familiar" with us and their answers can seem very insightful. These spirits will become more common as the spiritual darkness increases in these last days.

Reincarnation and Karma

These two teachings come from Hinduism, but they have been used a great deal in witchcraft as a way to understand the afterlife and consequences for sin. The belief of reincarnation teaches that once a person dies, they will assume a new body better or worse than the one they had before. Basically, reincarnation is an endless cycle of living and dying until one is perfected. What body a person gets in their next life depends on how they lived. The word karma describes what kind of reward one will receive in the next life or even in this present life. The problem with both beliefs is that they are unbiblical. We are not continually dying and living again for centuries. We live one life and then die at which point our soul will return to God where we will be judged (Hebrews 9:27). If we trusted in Jesus Christ and were faithful to Him, we will go to heaven, but if we rejected Jesus Christ and lived a sinful life we will end up in hell. Fortunately, we don't have to live under the punishment of the false belief of karma because Jesus Christ forgives all our sins and curses are broken in Jesus name. Under these false beliefs of reincarnation and karma people lead lives living under condemnation and see no possibility of change until their next life. Through Jesus Christ we can change our lives and live prosperously and peacefully. We can live an abundant and blessed life free from the fear of judgement!

Pagan Holidays

There are certain holidays people who live in the West practise. They are Easter, Christmas etc. These holidays have a lot of pagan elements incorporated into them and their chosen dates of celebration are pagan in origin. For example, Christmas is celebrated near the Winter Solstice taking place December 21-22. On this holiday people decorate trees with ornaments and set cookies and milk out at night for a jolly fellow who travels about the earth on Christmas Eve delivering presents. A lot of this is superstition and has no basis in the Bible. I'm not saying Christmas can't or shouldn't be practised but try to avoid the pagan elements. I believe the pagan elements of Christmas allow demons to come into many communities and households. This is the reason for the high level of depression and suicide during the Christmas season. Its not only being lonely, but a spiritually oppressive time. I personally believe that the real meaning of Christmas has been lost by many and become more demonic in nature. We must bring Jesus Christ back into Christmas and stop overemphasizing the pagan elements that have infiltrated this day/season. Likewise, Easter has some pagan elements incorporated into it. The Easter holiday is accompanied with watching the sun rise and Easter egg hunts. Watching the sun rise is basically about sun worship and has nothing to do with the resurrection of Jesus Christ. The Easter eggs have more to do with a fertility goddess and the celebration of spring than Jesus Christ.

Some people reading this book may have left a cult or pagan belief system but find themselves being invited to attend pagan holidays yearly by family or friends. Do not attend these festivals because you will bring yourself under a demonic influence. This does not mean you cannot associate with these people any longer, but we cannot practise these demonic holidays.

And what agreement has the temple of God with idols? For you are the temple of the living God. As God has said: "I will dwell in them and walk among them. I will be their God, and they shall be My people." Therefore, "Come out from among them and be separate, says the Lord. Do not touch what is unclean, and I will receive you." "I will be a Father to you, and you shall be My sons and daughters, says the Lord Almighty."

2 Corinthians 6:16-18 NKJV

When we become Christians, we get a new Father. Our Heavenly Father loves us and does not want us to practise pagan customs anymore for we belong to Him now. Remember witchcraft involves manipulation and friends and family not happy with your decision to follow Jesus Christ may try to seduce you back into their coven/organization. Resist the urge to conform and be unashamed to tell them you can longer participate in their practices because you've chosen to follow Jesus Christ.

I hope this brief overview of contemporary witchcraft was helpful. My goal was not to teach you about witchcraft, but to inform you so you are forearmed and know what to avoid.

Before I conclude this chapter, I'd like to talk about how witchcraft is affecting our youth in this day and age. Many people have read the Harry Potter books, but don't know that J.K. Rowling's ideas for her books were drawn directly from sources about real witchcraft.[xxiv] These books have appealed to a young audience and some teachers think its great if their students are reading anything. Remember that a crowd in Paul's day was stirred up by the python spirit to demand he be judged. This crowd knew little to nothing about Paul, but were angry nonetheless. When Paul was going to prayer in Philippi the python spirit in the slave girl was trying to draw the crowds to Paul. This spirit of python is targeting the children today and wants to enslave them like the girl Paul faced. The python spirit has created a craze or hysteria over the Harry Potter books and millions of young people have devoured these books and want more. As in the days of Philippi till now the python spirit continues to demonstrate its ability to manipulate the masses.

Unfortunately, witchcraft is not treated like any other religion and is viewed as harmless and fun. But witchcraft is no laughing matter and it leads to a covenant with false gods. The Harry Potter book series has popularized witchcraft and brought it into the mainstream. Witchcraft used to be taboo, but no longer thanks to J.K. Rowling's Harry Potter book series. In fact, witches are capitalizing on this rabid interest in magic and setting up real schools of witchcraft. The goal of the Harry Potter books was no doubt an effort to bring witchcraft into the school system. I do not believe that was the author's idea, but the python spirit that influenced her writing. Its very hypocritical that some schools and governments have permitted the teaching of witchcraft at their schools, but it is happening.[xxv] They'll ban school prayer or any teaching on Genesis but permit the teaching of the nature worshipping religion of witchcraft.

How to Defeat Python

1. Stay Focused

When Paul and his companions came to Philippi, they began their ministry with prayer. This is how every region should be dealt with on first approach. Prayer is a shield from enemy attack and it gives us insight into what is holding a region in captivity. In the case of Philippi, a python spirit was controlling the place through divination. The python spirit was trying to draw the attention of the crowds to Paul and his companions. The python spirit was using this strategy to distract Paul and his companions from their ministry of prayer. When Paul and his friends would not be distracted by the crowds the python spirit in the slave girl resorted to harassing Paul and his companions and constantly crying out after them.

Now it happened, as we went to prayer, that a certain slave girl possessed with a spirit of divination met us, who brought her masters much profit by fortune-telling. This girl followed Paul and us, and cried out, saying, "These men are the servants of the Most High God, who proclaim to us the way of salvation." And this she did for many days. But at midnight Paul and Silas were praying and singing hymns to God, and the prisoners were listening to them.

Acts 16:16-18, 25 NKJV

I put the verses from Acts 16 here to remind you of the story in case you forgot it. Paul and his companions are introduced to us as going to prayer, but after their arrest they are praying in jail! These guys are consistent and don't let their misfortune deter them from their calling and purpose in Philippi. In this case Paul and his friends were called to pray. Paul and Silas resisted the urge to be distracted by feelings of self-pity and depression and continued their prayer ministry.

2. Be Very Firm and Take Authority!

Paul was very patient with the slave girl, but he was also very forceful when dealing with this spirit. One must be firm with a python/divination spirit and be unyielding and resolute in dealing with it for it is a spirit of rebellion.

For rebellion is like the sin of divination, and arrogance is like the evil of idolatry.

1 Samuel 15:23a NIV

One thing I have noticed about rebellious people is that they are always testing those in authority and looking for weakness and compromise. They can sense those who are weak in their resolve or stressed. Therefore, one must be extremely vigilant with this kind of spirit. Rebellious people can be annoying and at times make us feel tired or weak. This is the witchcraft coming from this spirit trying to weaken us. Sometimes we'll have to get angry and absolutely crush this spirit by binding or casting it out in Jesus name!

But Paul, greatly annoyed, turned and said to the spirit, "I command you in the name of Jesus Christ to come out of her." And he came out that very hour.

Acts 16:18b NKJV

3. Become a Servant or Slave to God

Many come into battle with the python spirit and try to take authority over it only to be beaten up badly. We cannot bind a python spirit effectively if our lives are not submitted to God. I purposely emphasized the need for radical obedience in this book because the spirit of python has his slaves and if we are not slaves/servants to God like Paul we will be no match for python. The python spirit is a false authority, but if we are not submitted to the true authority of Jesus Christ our authority over the python spirit will not be very strong for without obedience to God our authority will be false also.

Therefore submit to God. Resist the devil and he will flee from you.

James 4:7 NKJV

4. Be on Fire for Jesus!

Paul and Silas never stopped praying to and worshipping God. Even when they were in that cold jail they continued to burn and shine brightly in the darkness. The python spirit wants to use the trials in our life to cause us to become bitter and cold with God. We must not lose our love for Jesus Christ even in the darkest of times. The python spirit wants to squeeze us until we can't breathe. Fire needs oxygen to burn and without the Holy Spirit we can't burn. We need to be continually filled with the Holy Spirit and be on fire. If we only manage to be lukewarm for Jesus Christ, we might become the prey of a python spirit. The python snake can detect the warmth of prey nearby. A lukewarm Christian will register enough heat to alert a python, but Python is not afraid of lukewarm Christians. Its afraid of Christians who are too hot to handle and will burn them. The python spirit cares not for cold Christians and unbelievers who are dead. It is on the hunt for those that are beginning to love and pursue God. The python spirit will watch these Christians until they cool off some and become lukewarm before deciding to strike. The only way to keep the python spirit permanently at bay is to be on fire for Jesus at all times.

"I know your works, that you are neither cold nor hot. I could wish you were cold or hot. So then, because you are lukewarm, and neither cold nor hot, I will vomit you out of My mouth.

Revelation 3:15-16 NKJV

5. Remain Confident in the Work God is Doing in Your Life

When one comes under an attack by a python spirit, they can feel tired and hopeless. Everything can appear dark and gloomy in the present, but we can't forget about our future. The python spirit wants us to be caught up in self-pity and pre-occupied with ourselves. We need to remember to hope in God and be confident He will finish the work He began in us.

Being confident of this very thing, that He who has begun a good work in you will complete it until the day of Jesus Christ;

Philippians 1:6 NKJV

We all have a calling from God and we need to remember that God wants to finish this work in our lives He called us to do.

6. Turn on the Lights

I believe happiness is something we choose to have. Its an attitude and not something that happens to us. When Paul and Silas were stuck in the jail, they chose to remain joyful and trusted in God. I also believe our level of joy is related to how much faith we have in God. We must decide to be joyful and not join in the despair that darkens the minds of many.

"Arise, shine, for your light has come, and the glory of the Lord rises upon you. See, darkness covers the

earth and thick darkness is over the peoples, but the Lord rises upon you and his glory appears over you. Nations will come to your light, and kings to the brightness of your dawn.

Isaiah 60:1-3 NIV

Do you want to be a leader or follower? I hope your answer is a leader. The world is a dark place and has little hope. God commands us to arise from our depression and shine. When the Church begins to shine with their hope in Jesus Christ the world will take note. We are not looking towards the end of the world or the anti-Christ, but the second coming of Jesus Christ. Its not all gloom and doom. When we start to shine kings and nations will see it and be inspired. Never stop fighting. If you turn the lights on people will come to you and ask you why you are so joyful. The python spirit wants us to quit on our kings, nations and the earth, but this is all a strategy to keep the world in darkness. Ignore Python's doom and gloom prophets and lead with hope!

7. Engage in Spiritual Warfare

Like Paul we can cast out the lesser spirits of python from ourselves and others. We can also bind the python spirit. Remember you are seated in heavenly places with Christ Jesus and can attack these python spirits like an eagle would. You are not subject to python it is subject to you. Never allow this spirit to set the terms of war. Take the initiative and kill the python spirit!

Renunciation of the Occult

I renounce all involvement in witchcraft I have practised by myself or with others. I renounce all forms of divination such as palm reading, tarot cards, astrology, rune stones, Ouija boards, seances, scrying, crystal balls, channeling, numerology, ESP, clairvoyance, fortune telling, soothsaying and other forms of divination. I also renounce sorcery, the contact of fairies or spirit guides, contacting or interacting with dragons, astral travel, meditation, wizardry, drawing on or manipulating energy, signs of the zodiac (renounce sign you believe you were born under), pagan observances or holidays, superstitions, idolatry, worship of false gods, mythology and all forms of false power. I renounce all these things and any demons connected to the activities in the name of Jesus Christ!

Prayer of Repentance for Rebellion

I repent for disobeying or cursing any legitimate government in my present or past. I repent for dishonoring and mocking the leaders or government figures God has placed in my life. I repent for trying to usurp or undermine my husband's authority (for women). I repent for trying to occupy an office God has not called me to like the pastorate (for women). I repent for disobeying my father and mother or cursing them. I repent for rebelling against or grieving any teachers in my life including teachers in the Church or the school system. I repent for challenging the police, fighting with or resisting the police, dishonoring or cursing the police. I repent for any dishonor of army veterans or active army personnel. I repent for any dishonor of the elderly. I repent for cursing God at anytime or for blatantly rejecting God's commands at anytime.

Binding Prayer for Python and Related Spirits

I bind every demon of python, witchcraft, divination, sorcery, narcotics, crystal meth, cocaine, heroin, marijuana, speed, alcohol, smoking, addiction, rebellion, disobedience, stubborn, self-will, stiff-necked, defiance, depression, hopelessness, despair, suicide and death.

Note: This is by no means an exhaustive list, so you can add or remove demons you wish to bind at your leisure.

Prayer of Self-Deliverance from Python and Related Spirits

I command every demon of python, witchcraft, divination, sorcery, fortune telling, soothsaying, clairvoyance, astrology, palm reading, Ouija board, séance, channeling, spirit guide, haunting, ghosts, horror movies, curses, blasphemy, numerology, chiromancy, totem animal, crystal energy, energy, manipulation, Satanism, coven, oaths, secrets, magic, eastern mysticism, meditation, false light, rebellion, disobedience, defiance, stubbornness, idolatry, lawlessness, anti-Christ, 666, hopelessness, despair, burnout, exhaustion, constriction, depression, suicide, insomnia, anxiety, panic attack, bipolar, addiction, slavery, bondage, broken spirit, crushed dreams, broken heart to come out of me now in the name of Jesus Christ. You demons can never return to me at anytime in the future nor can you transfer to any friends or family of mine. You are banished completely from my life and must go to the pit right now in the name of Jesus Christ!

Note: You can add or remove any demons from the prayer above at your leisure. This is a suggested prayer and it is by no means exhaustive in nature.

Powerful Words Given to the Church of Philippi for Overcoming Python

Being confident of this, that he who began a good work in you will carry it on to completion until the day of Christ Jesus.

Philippians 1:6 NIV

I hope you never have to face Python, but if you do these verses given to the Church of Philippi will give you victory! When Python enters our life, it is usually to stall the work of God in our lives. There are times we can feel forgotten by God and despair. When Paul and his companions were going to prayer, they were encountered by the slave girl with the python spirit and harassed. This encounter did not happen once, but for many days. This was a campaign of harassment by Python that was meant to break them with discouragement and compel them to leave Philippi. Paul had enough and cast Python out of the slave girl. This resulted in the slave masters becoming angry and they stirred up a mob demanding that the magistrates imprison Paul and Silas. Paul and Silas could've sunk into a deep depression because of days of harassment and their imprisonment. But instead of discouragement they began to pray and worship. I believe they were able to do this because of what was written in Philippians 1:6 which I posted above. Paul and Silas weren't broken because they had confidence in Jesus Christ and knew He still had a purpose and plan for them. We must hold on to the hope we have in Jesus Christ and remember any prophecy concerning our calling (s).

For to me, to live is Christ and to die is gain.

Philippians 1:21 NIV

Python wants us to fear loss. The above verse shows us that we can be free of this fear by making Jesus Christ our greatest desire. If Jesus is our greatest desire any loss of the material and otherwise will not impact us like Python would like. To be fearless of loss or death will make us almost invincible! When Jesus Christ is everything to us, we will want nothing, nor will we fear anything else.

Do nothing out of selfish ambition or vain conceit. Rather, in humility value others above yourselves.

Philippians 2:3 NIV

Remember Python loves a crowd and he will either try to destroy us through fame or public infamy. Don't be manipulated Python's use of public opinion. This reminds me of how the Fake News were all wrong about Hillary winning the election in 2016. Donald Trump won the election and proved everyone wrong! Pray for President Trump for Python is still trying to use public opinion to manipulate President Trump. Python knows Trump likes fame. Pray President Trump is free from the lust for fame and that he would decide to do the right thing at every occasion.

Rejoice in the Lord always. I will say it again: Rejoice! Let your gentleness be evident to all. The Lord is near. Do not be anxious about anything, but in every situation, by prayer and petition, with thanksgiving, present your requests to God. And the peace of God, which transcends all understanding, will guard your hearts and your minds in Christ Jesus. Finally, brothers and sisters, whatever is true, whatever is noble, whatever is right, whatever is pure, whatever is

lovely, whatever is admirable—if anything is excellent or praiseworthy—think about such things. Whatever you have learned or received or heard from me, or seen in me—put it into practice. And the God of peace will be with you.

Philippians 4:4-9 NIV

I believe Paul is instructing us in the above verses that peace and joy can only be found in healthy habits. Paul tells us we must decide to rejoice. We often think joy is found in everything going our way in a day or popping a happy pill. The joy that comes through outward experiences is temporary. Permanent joy can only be a reality when we decide to rejoice in the Lord always. Our joy can only be found in our Lord Jesus Christ. If we are looking to other things for our joy our joy will be short lived. Paul also instructs us to continually pray in every situation. Anxiety can be a persistent adversary so one must be persistent in prayer. When we remember to add thanks to our prayers, we will see the peace of God entering our lives. Thanksgiving reminds not only God, but us of God's faithfulness. When we remember His goodness towards us and His unfailing acts of kindness our faith in Him increases. As our faith increases our trust in Jesus Christ builds. This trust brings the calming peace of God into our lives so that we are guarded in heart and mind. We will feel secure. Finally, Paul encourages us to watch our thought life. Watching the news for several hours each day will not bring us peace, but the fear and discouragement Python is proclaiming through his false prophets/journalists. We become what we focus on. Paul encourages us to think about things that are praiseworthy. Would Jesus Christ approve of what we are thinking about? Do our thoughts line up with God's Word or the Bible? We must be careful with what we think about. This will determine whether we have the peace of God or not.

I know what it is to be in need, and I know what it is to have plenty. I have learned the secret of being content in any and every situation, whether well fed or hungry, whether living in plenty or in want. I can do all this through him who gives me strength.

Philippians 4:12-13 NIV

I wonder if Paul was reflecting on his time in the jail of Philippi when he wrote the above verses. Paul talks about the secret of being content in any and every situation and attributes it to Jesus Christ who gives him strength. Paul is certain that he can do all things with the strength of Jesus Christ working through him. This is a powerful secret and necessary for survival. Many find themselves in literal prisons or prisons of the mind. These prisons can leave us feeling vulnerable, plundered and helpless. But this is different when we make Jesus Christ our source for all things.

These verses from the letter to the Philippians gives us insight into how to defeat Python. Python wants us to seek fame or fear becoming infamous. When these tactics fail, he will try to make us depressed and anxious. He wants to remind us of what we lost. But Python can never take Jesus Christ from us and the freedom we seek can only be found in Jesus Christ. Jesus Christ is the key to our prison door and our way out!

Donald Trump the Destroyer

There has never been a man in American politics who has caused so much polarization as President Donald Trump. Of course, this polarization is primarily rooted in America's policy with Israel and not with President Trump alone. Before President Trump came into office America was already a very divided place. Many want to blame this man for the present divide in the nation, but they are looking in the wrong place. The United States of America has been trying to create an Israel and Palestine alongside each other for some time. Unfortunately, the U.S. has been warned many times not to attempt dividing Israel, but they have persisted.

I will gather all nations and bring them down to the Valley of Jehoshaphat. There I will put them on trial for what they did to my inheritance, my people Israel, because they scattered my people among the nations and divided up my land.

Joel 3:2 NIV

The Lord had said to Abram, "Go from your country, your people and your father's household to the land I will show. "I will make you into a great nation, and I will bless you; I will make your name great, and you will be a blessing. I will bless those who bless you, and whoever curses you I will curse; and all peoples on earth will be blessed through you."

Genesis 12:1-3 NIV

You may be wondering what Donald Trump and Israel have to do with this book and the python spirit at this moment. Glad you asked. I will reveal the answer in a moment.

The United States and the world are at a critical juncture and much of this has to do with how President Trump deals with Israel. I know many who read that will reflexively come to the defense of President Trump and insist he is a strong supporter of Israel. It is true that President Trump designated Jerusalem as the capital of Israel and moved the embassy there, but in that same speech he mentioned that the borders of Jerusalem and Israel were still subject to final status negotiations.[xxvi] President Trump later informed the public that he supported a two-state solution on Israel on September 26, 2018.[xxvii] After President Trump made this announcement he unknowingly opened the gates of hell into the United States. The United States is on the verge of destruction and this has been made possible by President Trump's strong connection with the python spirit aka Apollo. This connection is most evident at his penthouse in New York City where he has more than one painting of Apollo decorating his living space.[xxviii] Remember Apollo's name means "destroyer".

They had as king over them the angel of the Abyss, whose name in Hebrew is Abaddon and in Greek is Apollyon (that is Destroyer).

Revelation 9:11 NIV

Interestingly, this isn't wild speculation on my part that President Trump is associated with destruction as many have used the moniker or nickname "Destroyer" to describe President Trump. One of the many examples I can use is that of Kim Jong Un calling President Trump a "destroyer".[xxix] This may not seem unusual as many words have been exchanged between President Trump and Kim Jong Un of North Korea, but another leader in running for the Chancellery of Germany also called President Trump a destroyer.[xxx] Any search on the internet will reveal that many media outlets see President Trump as a "destroyer". It is ironic that President Trump who built a real estate empire has become known to many as a destroyer.

I believe President Trump as a leader could lead the U.S. and the world into a great era of freedom and prosperity. But this will require the people of the U.S. and those nations knowing Jesus Christ turning back to Him. Those nations that know Jesus Christ I am referring to are Canada, the nations of Europe and Australia along with New Zealand. While it is true the U.S. along with these other nations have gone astray there is without a doubt a memory and knowledge of the Bible and Jesus Christ which cannot be ignored.

After all, there has been a culture war that has been happening for decades now and it hasn't been resolved because the Church in the West has not surrendered to the apostate forces at work in their societies. The battles over abortion, the legalization of gay marriage, transgenderism, drugs and other causes will continue. Fortunately, there is hope for Christians as President Trump has had the privilege of shifting the U.S. Supreme Court to the right. He has appointed two new U.S. Supreme Court justices Neil Gorsuch and Brett Kavanaugh. This has infuriated the left in the U.S. and the world as they watch their power over this high court being destroyed. There is a great deal of destruction coming to international organizations as well. President Trump trashed NAFTA which was not favorable to the U.S. and created the new USMCA which apparently puts America first. President Trump also withdrew the U.S. from the TPP (Trans Pacific Partnership) leaving a gaping hole there. In addition, President Trump has encouraged the United Kingdom to continue its push to separate from Europe through BREXIT. President Trump has also suggested that France leave the European Union for a better trade deal with the U.S. This interference from President Trump in the affairs of the European Union is angering many and is beginning to result in a rift in NATO. The President of France Emmanuel Macron and the Chancellor of Germany Angela Merkel are both calling for a "European Army".[xxxi] President Macron even suggested that Europe needed to consider the U.S. as a military threat![xxxii]

Why is everything going bonkers like this? Well, President Trump is God's tool to destroy the international cabal or order and bring back nationalism. The world has been pursuing a path of peace without God. The same thing was done at the tower of Babel.

Now the whole world had one language and a common speech. As people moved eastward, they found a plain in Shinar and settled there. They said to each other, "Come, let's make bricks and bake them thoroughly." They used brick instead of stone, and tar for mortar. Then they said, "Come, let us build ourselves a city, with a tower that reaches to the heavens, so that we may make a name for ourselves; otherwise we will be scattered over the face of the whole earth." But the Lord came down to see the city and the tower the people were building. The Lord said, "If as one people speaking the same language they have begun to do this, then nothing they plan to do will be impossible for them. Come, let us go down and confuse their language so they will not understand each other." So the Lord scattered them from there over all the earth, and they stopped building the city. That is why it was called Babel— because there the Lord confused the language of the

whole world. From there the Lord scattered them over the face of the whole earth.

Genesis 11:1-9 NIV

Jesus Christ is using President Trump as His instrument to destroy the world order that has been building for some time. The U.N. will collapse along with many other international organizations for they have become a modern-day Tower of Babel. The world is in a state of confusion as the new world order is being destroyed. Many Christians are celebrating the collapse of the NWO, but while I believe this is good news, we must also pray that the U.S. and other nations aren't destroyed. Remember the python spirit/Apollo has a strong influence on President Trump and he could also destroy the U.S. if America does not repent and turn back to Jesus Christ. The world order that is presently being destroyed is headquartered in New York City. This is the city where President Trump dwells when he's not ruling in Washington D.C. It was in NYC where the World Trade Center towers fell. More destruction will come to NYC and America if they do not repent. Jesus Christ can and will use President Trump to destroy the U.S. if they decide not to repent of their sins. How will this happen you may ask?

My companion attacks his friends; he violates his covenant. His talk is smooth as butter, yet war is in his heart; his words are more soothing than oil, yet they are drawn swords.

Psalms 55:20-21 NIV

President Trump has shown he is able to change his mind at any moment. He has ended organizations and treaties that were formerly in place. Through Twitter and news conferences President Trump has been an instrument of division. President Trump is not one who unites, but divides. President Trump is at war with globalism and the Communist influences being uncovered in the U.S. and the world. President Trump has singled out ANTIFA a lawless anarchist group that protests on the streets using violent means. They are Communists who hate any return to Christianity. President Trump's words are incendiary and are creating a destructive atmosphere. The world will see another world war, but how severe it will be no one can really know. This world war has already started as President Trump has essentially declared a trade war with the world. Nations will become increasingly divided as Jesus Christ shakes all nations for their rebellion towards Him. Many have preached a cuddly false Jesus who never gets angry with sin. Time is up, and Jesus Christ is judging the earth. If the U.S. and other nations do not repent, they will be destroyed also. President Trump is the instrument of Jesus Christ's wrath. If anyone doubts Jesus Christ is angry, I would urge you to look at Malibu in Los Angeles County. A fire arose there that destroyed the homes of many who have been promoting sexual lust in the media and polluting the world. Miley Cyrus, Bruce

Jenner aka Kaitlyn Jenner, Lady Gaga, Robin Thicke and others who promoted sexual filth saw their homes burnt to ashes!

    I would like to conclude this chapter by encouraging you the reader. President Trump has not only been raised up to destroy, but to build up. The U.S. Supreme Court's shift to the right and the addition of two new justices by President Trump is an example of this. Before President Trump became president, he built buildings and a real estate empire. If the saints prevail in prayer this man will continue to help Jesus Christ and aid in the building of Christ's kingdom, however, if the saints do not prevail the python spirit/Apollo will gain influence and bring great destruction. This false god Apollo was known as an archer and this spirit wants to start a nuclear war through President Trump. He wants to unleash his arrows/missiles through President Trump so that many people die and go to hell. Like Jeremiah the prophet President Trump has been raised up to destroy and build. Let us have hope and pray to Jesus Christ so that He would bring repentance to the U.S. and the world in order that people and nations of the earth are not destroyed.

Then the Lord reached out his hand and touched my mouth and said to me, "I have put my words in your mouth. See, today I appoint you over nations and kingdoms to uproot and tear down, to destroy and overthrow, to build and to plant."

Jeremiah 1:9-10 NIV

[i] https://www.foxnews.com/science/florida-man-captures-mammoth-17-foot-python-sets-record
[ii] https://www.facebook.com/kyle.penniston/posts/2134635193234210
[iii] https://www.biblestudytools.com/blogs/matthew-s-harmon/the-city-of-philippi-in-the-bible.html
[iv] https://bible.org/article/christianity-best-thing-ever-happened-women
[v] https://www.persecution.com/
[vi] https://en.wikipedia.org/wiki/Philippi
[vii] http://fortune.com/2015/09/21/psychic-business-advice/
[viii] https://www.cnn.com/2018/09/26/politics/trump-israeli-palestinian/index.html
[ix] https://www.cnbc.com/2018/10/10/us-markets-bond-yields-and-data-in-focus.html
[x] https://www.usatoday.com/story/news/politics/2018/10/11/hurricane-michael-smashed-tyndall-key-air-base-homeland-defense/1601454002/
[xi] https://www.cnn.com/2018/10/27/us/synagogue-attack-suspect-robert-bowers-profile/index.html
[xii] https://www.nbcnews.com/news/us-news/free-speech-week-uc-berkeley-canceled-milo-yiannopoulos-blames-school-n804171
[xiii] https://www.dw.com/en/how-the-summer-of-love-came-to-san-francisco-50-years-ago/a-40236165
[xiv] https://en.wikipedia.org/wiki/LGBT_culture_in_San_Francisco
[xv] https://www.vox.com/2017/8/25/16189064/antifa-charlottesville-dc-unite-the-right-mark-bray
[xvi] http://officialproudboys.com/proud-boys/whoaretheproudboys/
[xvii] https://www.telegraph.co.uk/technology/facebook/10930654/Facebooks-71-gender-options-come-to-UK-users.html
[xviii] https://en.wikipedia.org/wiki/Incarceration_in_the_United_States
[xix] https://www.ncbi.nlm.nih.gov/pmc/articles/PMC4439707/
[xx] https://www.ncbi.nlm.nih.gov/pmc/articles/PMC4439707/
[xxi] http://www.shakmyth.org/myth/28/apollo/some+secondary+sources
[xxii] https://en.wikipedia.org/wiki/Hippocratic_Oath

[xxiii] https://classroom.synonym.com/greek-mythology-apollo-plague-21925.html
[xxiv] https://www.thoughtco.com/is-harry-potter-a-pagan-book-250154
[xxv] https://www.telegraph.co.uk/news/religion/9206178/Its-beyond-belief-to-teach-witchcraft.html
[xxvi] https://www.vox.com/world/2017/12/6/16741528/trump-jerusalem-speech-israel-tel-aviv
[xxvii] https://www.cnn.com/2018/09/26/politics/trump-israeli-palestinian/index.html
[xxviii] https://www.dailymail.co.uk/news/article-3303819/Inside-Donald-Trump-s-100m-penthouse-lots-marble-gold-rimmed-cups-son-s-toy-personalized-Mercedes-15-000-book-risqu-statues.html
[xxix] https://www.cnbc.com/2017/11/11/north-korea-says-trump-begged-for-a-war-during-his-asia-trip.html
[xxx] https://af.reuters.com/article/worldNews/idAFKBN18Q1JF
[xxxi] https://globalnews.ca/news/4660528/angela-merkel-european-army/
[xxxii] https://www.independent.co.uk/news/world/europe/emmanuel-macron-european-army-france-russia-us-military-defence-eu-a8619721.html

Made in the USA
Columbia, SC
25 July 2022